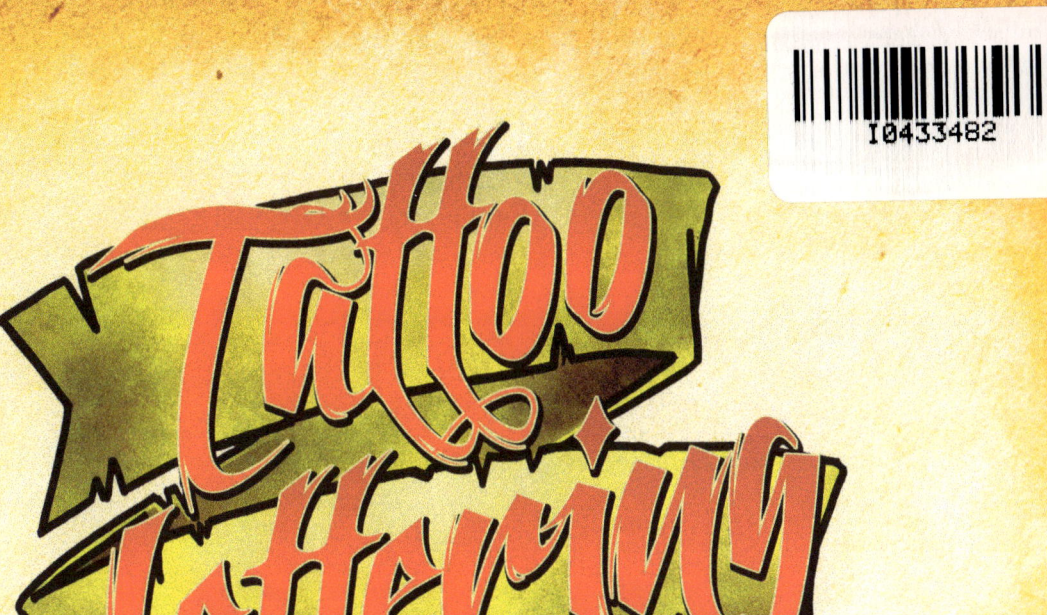

By Superior Tattoo

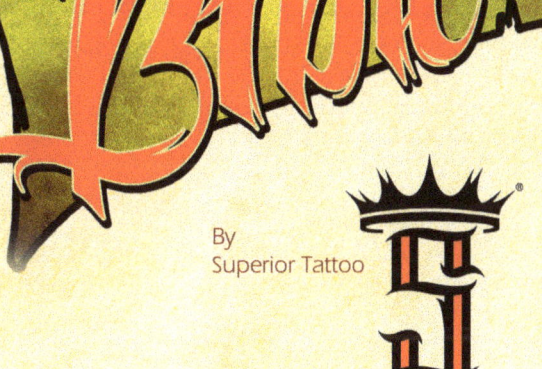

Legals

First published in 2014 by ArtKulture an imprint of
Wolfgang Publications Inc.,
PO Box 223, Stillwater MN 55082

© Superior Tattoo, 2014

All rights reserved. With the exception of quoting brief passages for the purposes of review no part of this publication may be reproduced without prior written permission from the publisher.

The information in this book is true and complete to the best of our knowledge. All recommendations are made without any guarantee on the part of the author or publisher, who also disclaim any liability incurred in connection with the use of this data or specific details.

We recognize that some words, model names and designations, for example, mentioned herein are the property of the trademark holder. We use them for identification purposes only. This is not an official publication. Wolfgang and ArtKulture control the book with the permission of Jim Watson and Cherie Watson. There are a few text changes in the front section and the last three pages, in this 2024 document.

ISBN-13: 978-1-935828-92-1

Printed and bound in U.S.A.

Acknowledgements

Superior Tattoo Equipment, Inc. would like to thank all the tattoo artists out there that continuously impress the world with their amazing abilities. For this specific book, we decided to focus specifically on Tattoo Lettering, which seems to grow more popular by each passing day. Whether you are doing a tribute tattoo, a meaningful quote, or a clean, simple loved one's name, just the right font can make all the difference. With Superior having the industry's largest flash library, we began to scour our collection to bring you the most complete, and eclectic lettering designs ever.

Over the years, we have collected many sheets of flash, and are thankful for each and every artist we have built relationships with throughout our existence. This book features lettering designs from Jim Watson, Bob Sims, Matthew Ratlief, Michael Tsatsopoulos, Jose Sauceda, Summer Henry, Samantha Shaw, Melody Cooper, Micah McCoubrey, and Lyle Norcott. We would like to thank these artists for their superior artwork, and dedication to distributing their ideas to struggling artists in need of help. We would also like to offer a very special "Thank You" to Tom Kaczor; without his dedication and extreme attention to detail, this book would never have been completed on time. If we missed anyone, we apologize from the bottom of our hearts. You are what make the tattoo industry one of the most fun and most rewarding industries to work in.

Superior Tattoo Equipment would also like to add a special "Thank You" to Timothy Remus and Jacki Mitchell at Wolfgang Publications. Time and time again as these books are published, they go above and beyond the call of duty. Their dedication to publishing and getting Superior Tattoo's artwork into the hands of artists worldwide is palpable. What they are able to do with our designs, and the amount of distributors Wolfgang has access to is incredible, and we look forward to expanding our line of books with them in the future.

Thank you and enjoy the book!

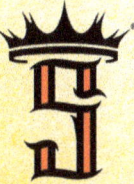

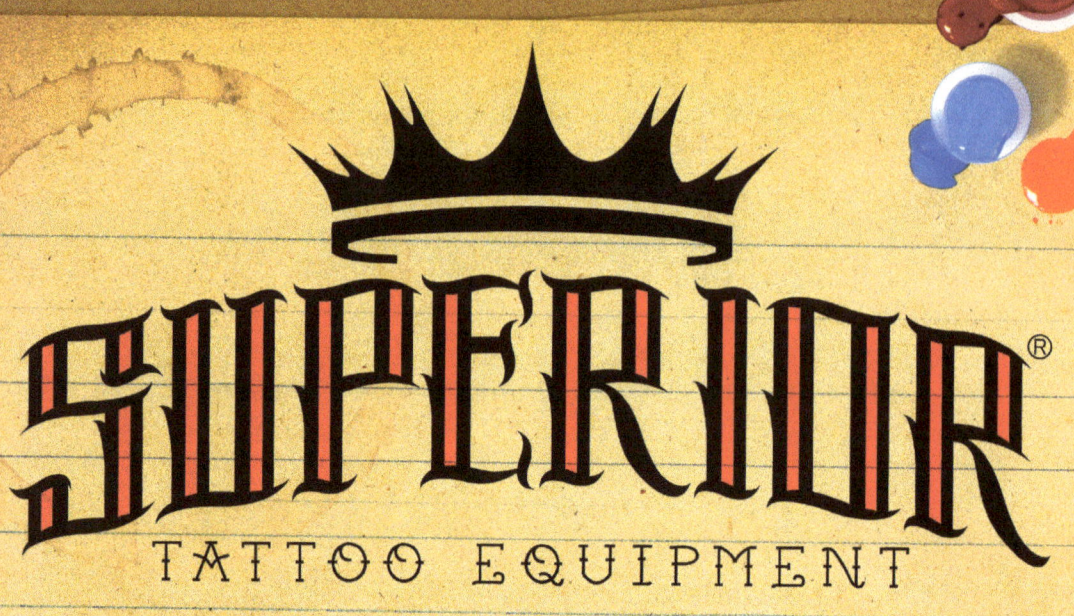

SUPERIOR
TATTOO EQUIPMENT

Since 1991, Superior Tattoo Equipment, Inc. has been serving the tattoo industry by offering supplies that are essential to the tattoo community at low, affordable prices. Through hard work, employee dedication, premium products and low prices Superior has not only survived in this industry, but has grown to become one of its most recognizable brands. Superior Tattoo has grown to be America's #1 supplier and has many claims to fame, with patents on several inventions, the largest tattoo flash library available, and the best selection of tattoo kits to both start new careers and continue fulfilling the needs of the seasoned artist. Superior Tattoo Equipment is in constant communication with tattoo professionals all over the world, gathering feedback to make our products the very best in the industry and available at prices everyone can afford. Superior hand-builds many of the tattoo machines they carry in their warehouse, in Phoenix, Arizona. From winding their own coils to hand assembling machines daily, Superior takes pride in using local suppliers for parts and merchandise when possible.

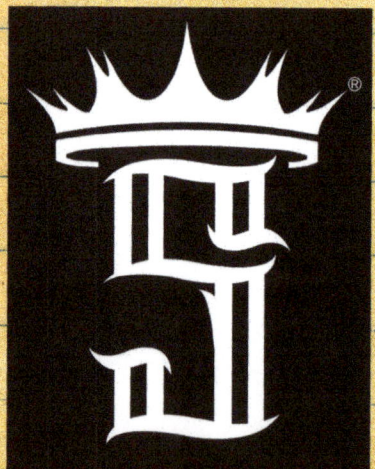

As an industry leader, Superior Tattoo knows that quick turnaround on orders is one of the major things that set them apart from their competition. Their physical store in Phoenix is open 7 days a week, while internet and phone-in orders can be placed 24 hours a day. When an artist needs a product, and needs it fast, Superior is the only choice!

Superior Tattoo's website is up-to-date, secure, and filled with everything you need to start tattooing. New products are added to inventory daily, the moment they are available. Superior's website is updated every day, who else can make that claim? Buying tattoo equipment shouldn't be intimadating, and Superior has made it as stress-free as possible!

From the Publisher

It all started in 2009 when Jim Watson called me, and asked if we could make a book from of their collection of flash art. Obviously, I said yes and we put together the Tattoo Bible Book One, followed by the Two and Three Bibles (all three are still available). More Tattoo books came along, thanks to the crew at Superior Tattoo Equipment. The Man really made all those books happened – including his own - Jim Watson's Tattoo Sketchbook.

At Wolfgang, we've been publishing books for thirty years and during that time, we've had publishing partners and authors that run the gamut from terrific to terrible. Superior Tattoo and Jim Watson definitely falls into the terrific category. Not only were they professional in all their dealings with us, they were simply easy to get along with, and never exhibit any attitude during discussions about current and future titles. And even though Jim has moved to Tattoo heaven, and the crew has scattered to shops all over the country, we need to thank all the members of the team – especially Tom Kaczor - for the hard work and for consistently sending all the materials in on time and very well organized.

One more note: I left the Superior Tattoo Equipment info (page 4) in the book, simply because it tells the world that the Superior was a foundation of the Tattoo Industry with their improved tools, the soothing products for the after-tattoo, and the books.

Timothy Remus

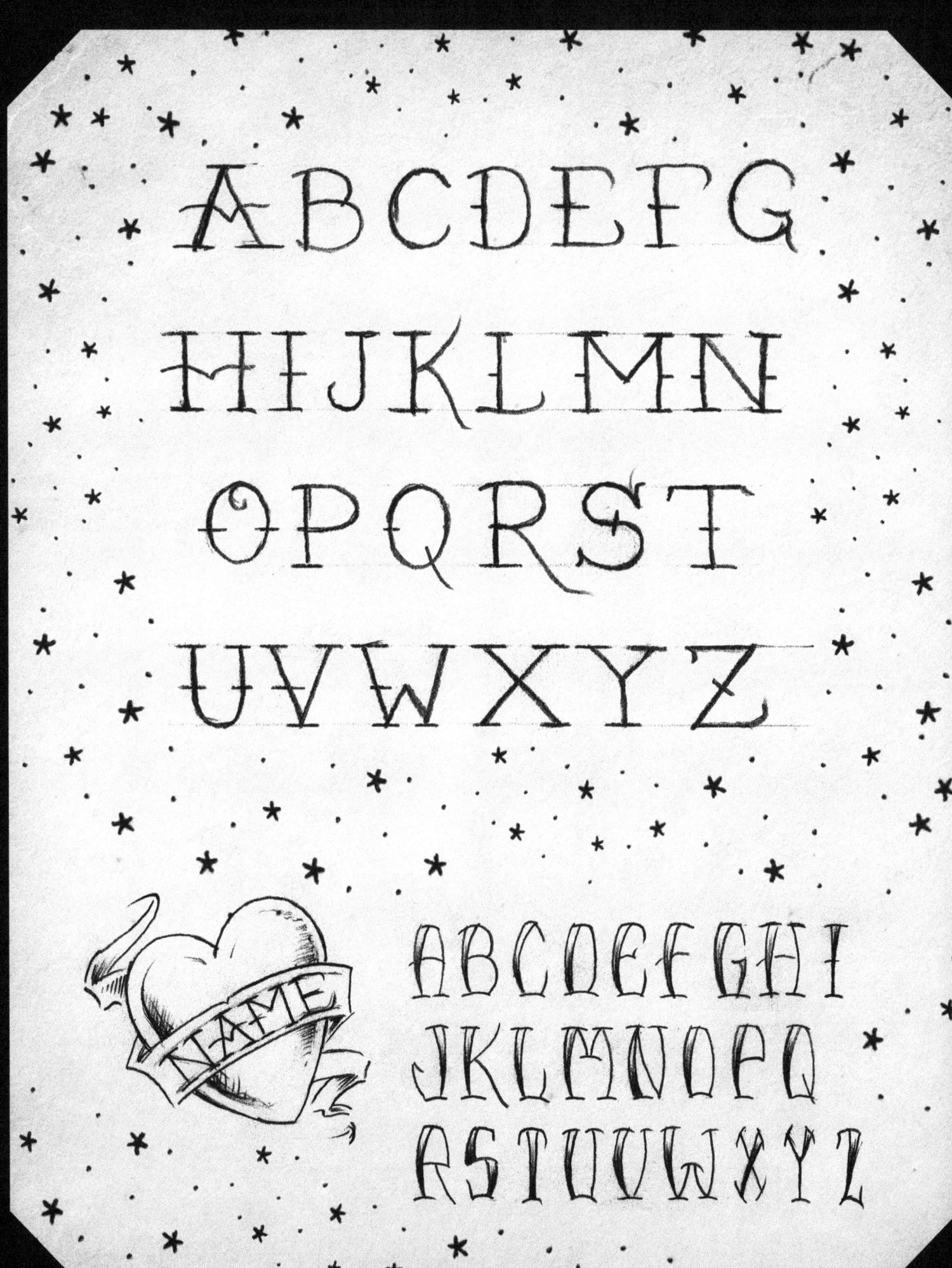

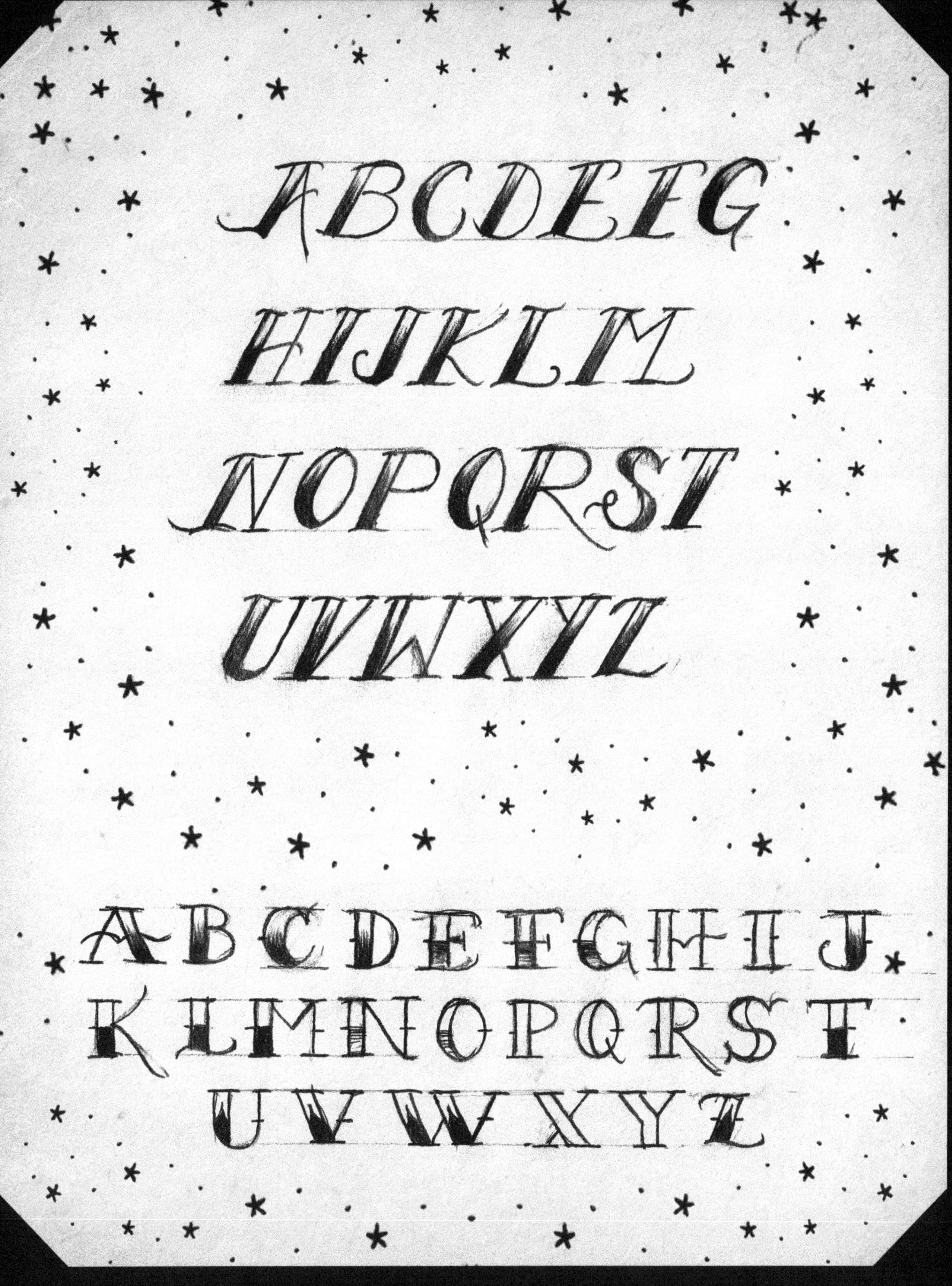

ABCDEFG
HIJKLM
NOPQRST
UVWXYZ

ABCDEFGHIJ
KLMNOPQRST
UVWXYZ

ABCDEFGH
JKLMNOPQ
RSTUVWXY

ABCDEFG
HIJKLMN
OPQRST
UVWXYZ

Dream

Dream

Dream

Dream

Dream

Dream

Forever Young

Forever Young

Forever Young

Forever Young

Forever Young

Forever Young

ABCDEFG
HIJKLMN
OPQRSTU
VWXYZ

abcdefg
hijklmno
pqrstuvw
xyz

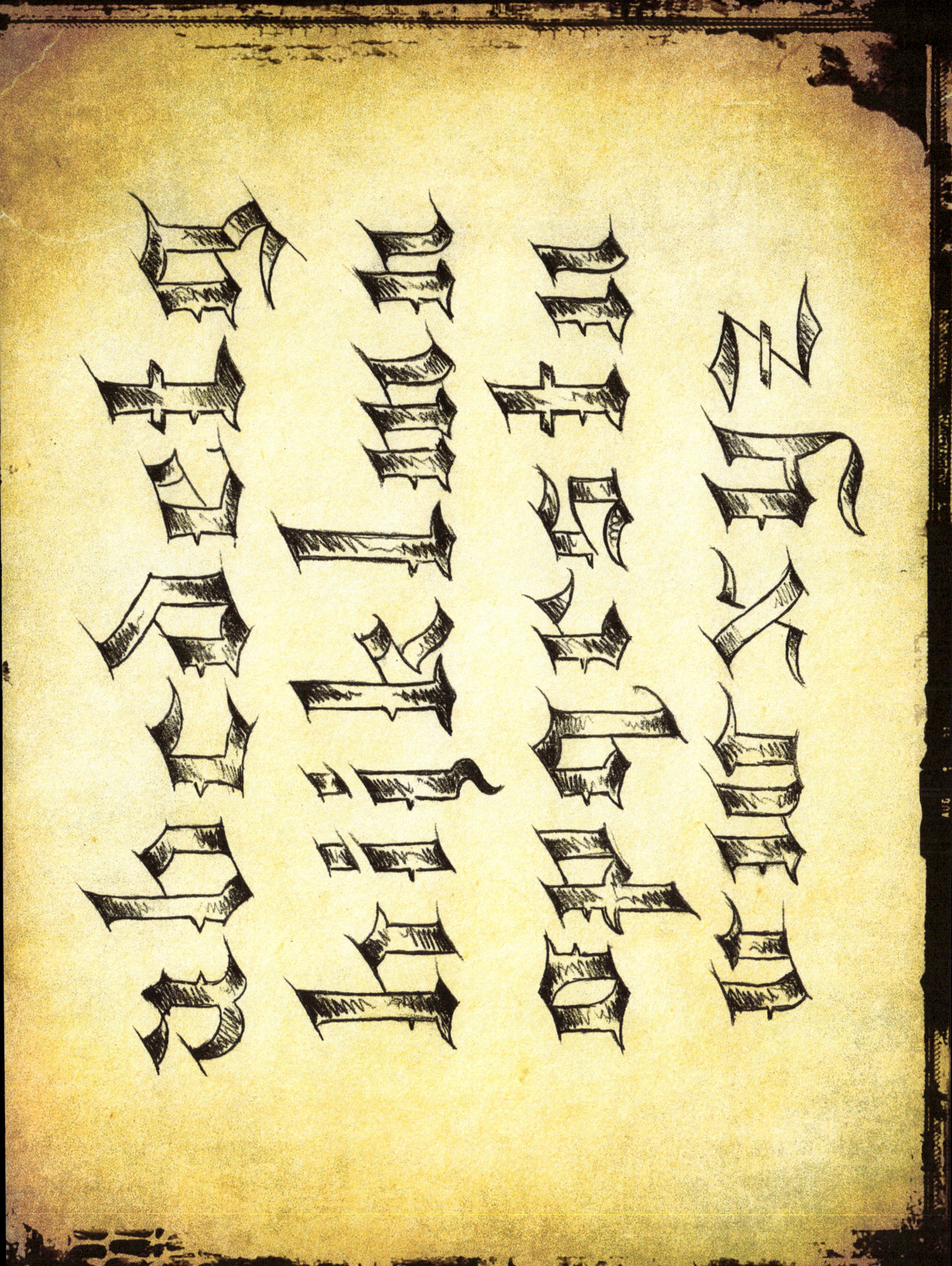

A B C D

E F G H

I J K L

M N O P

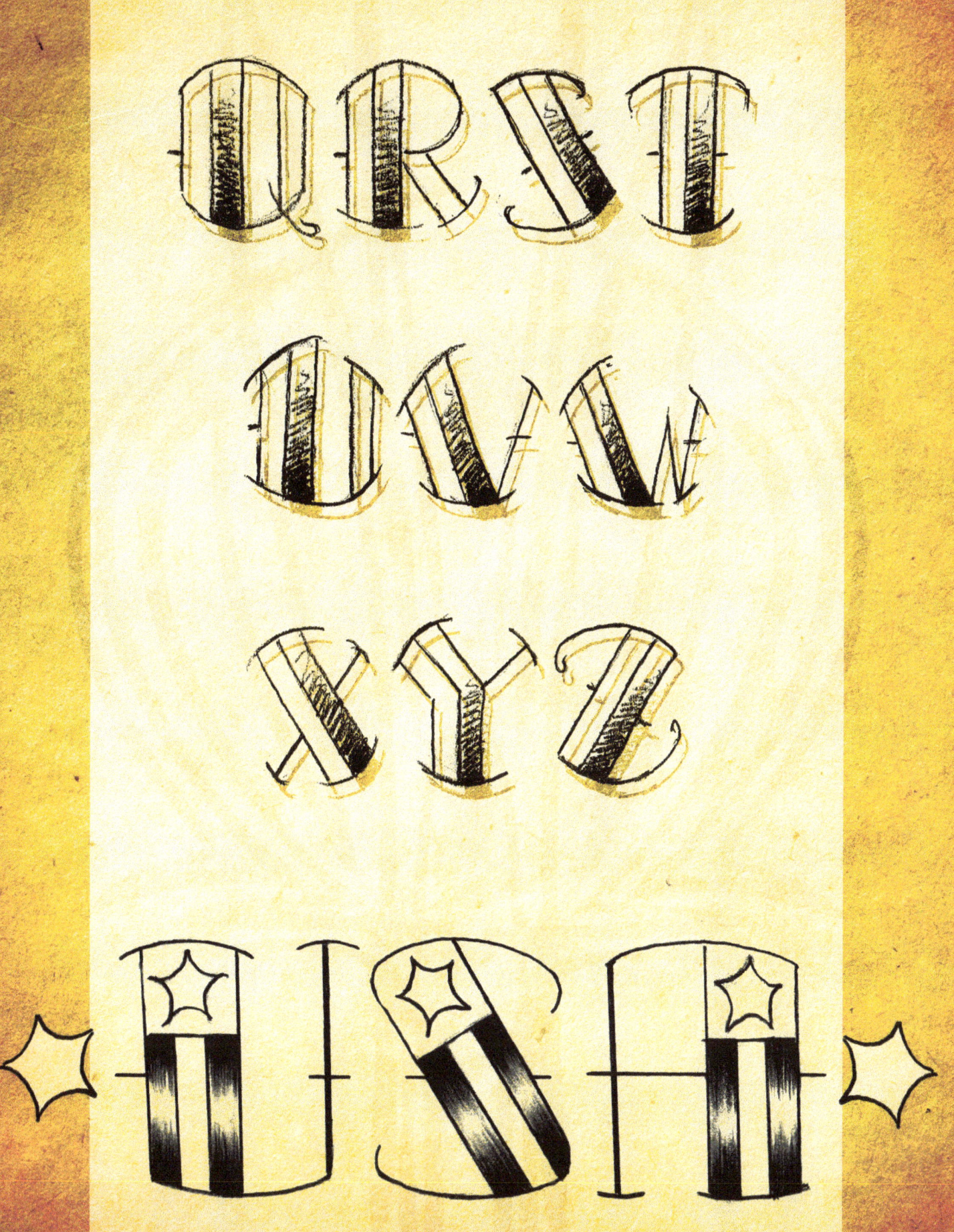

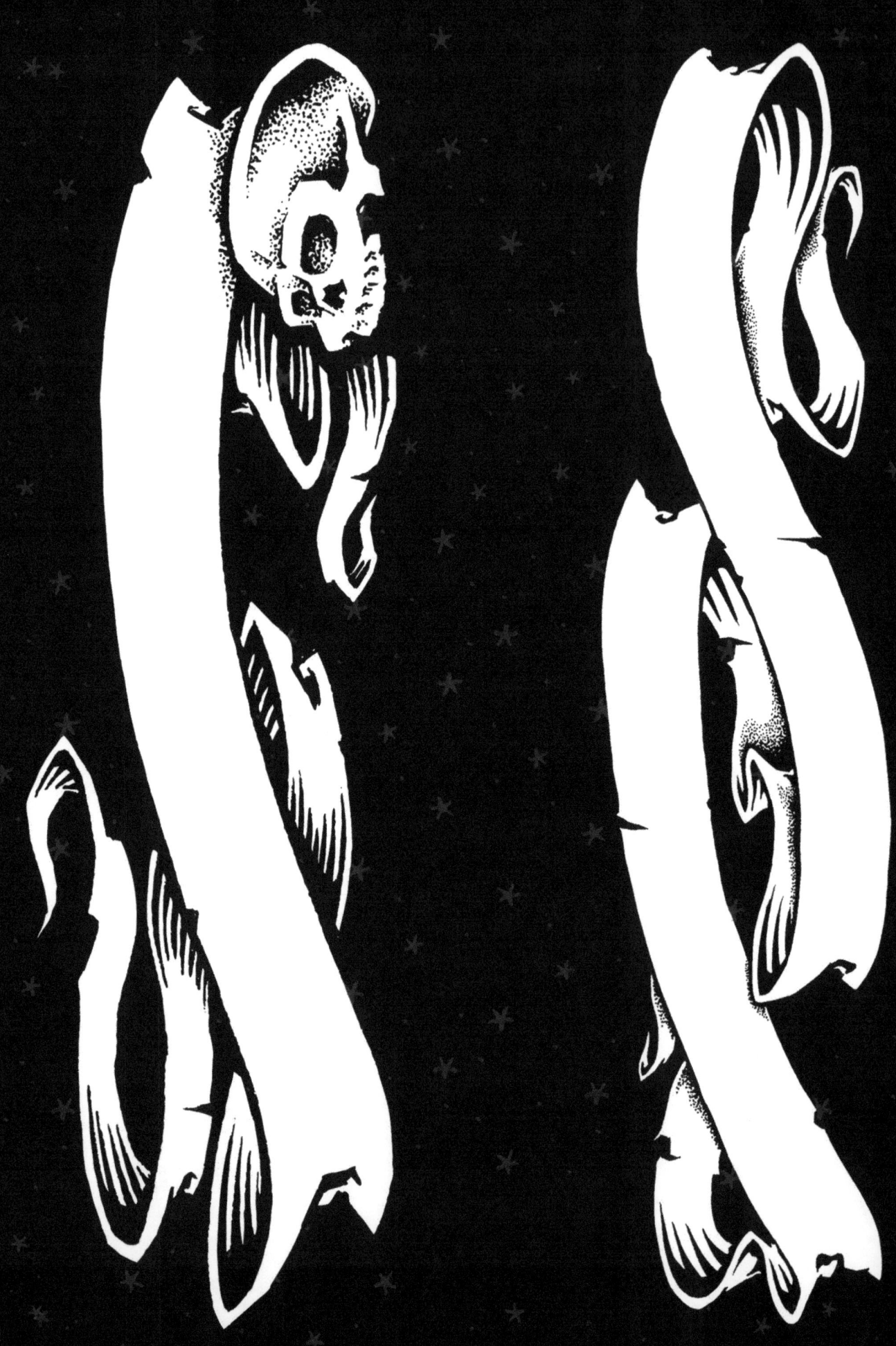

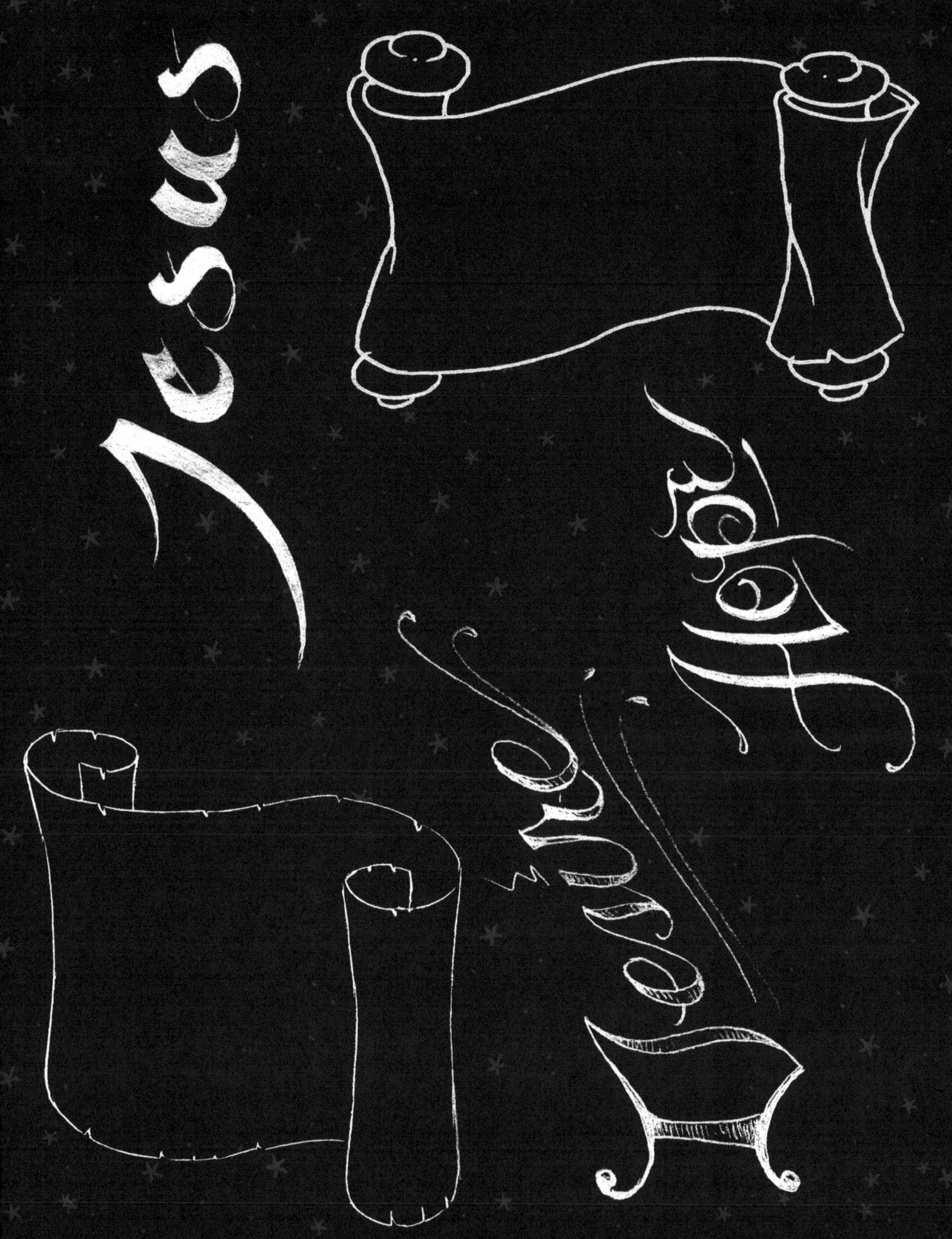

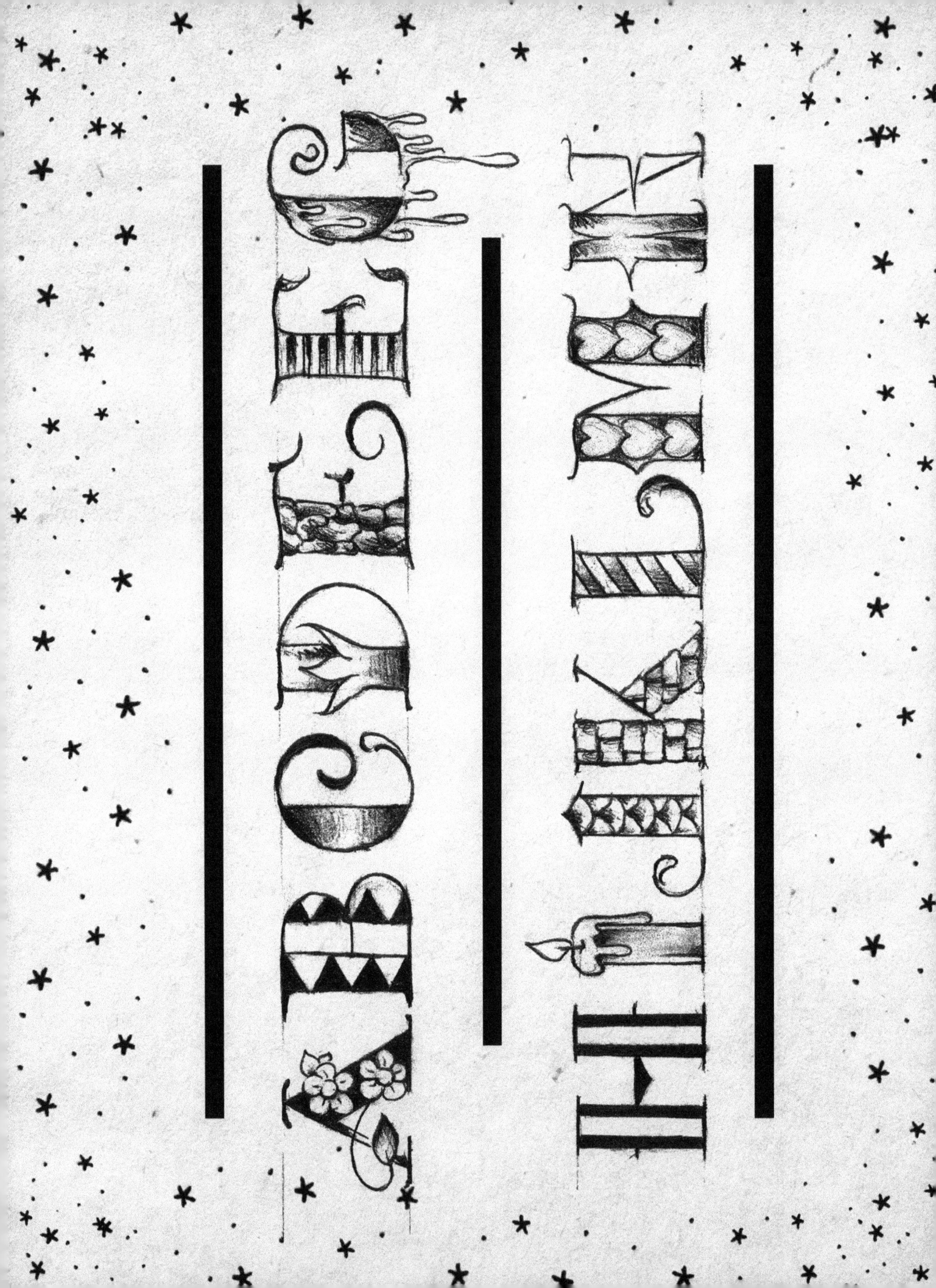

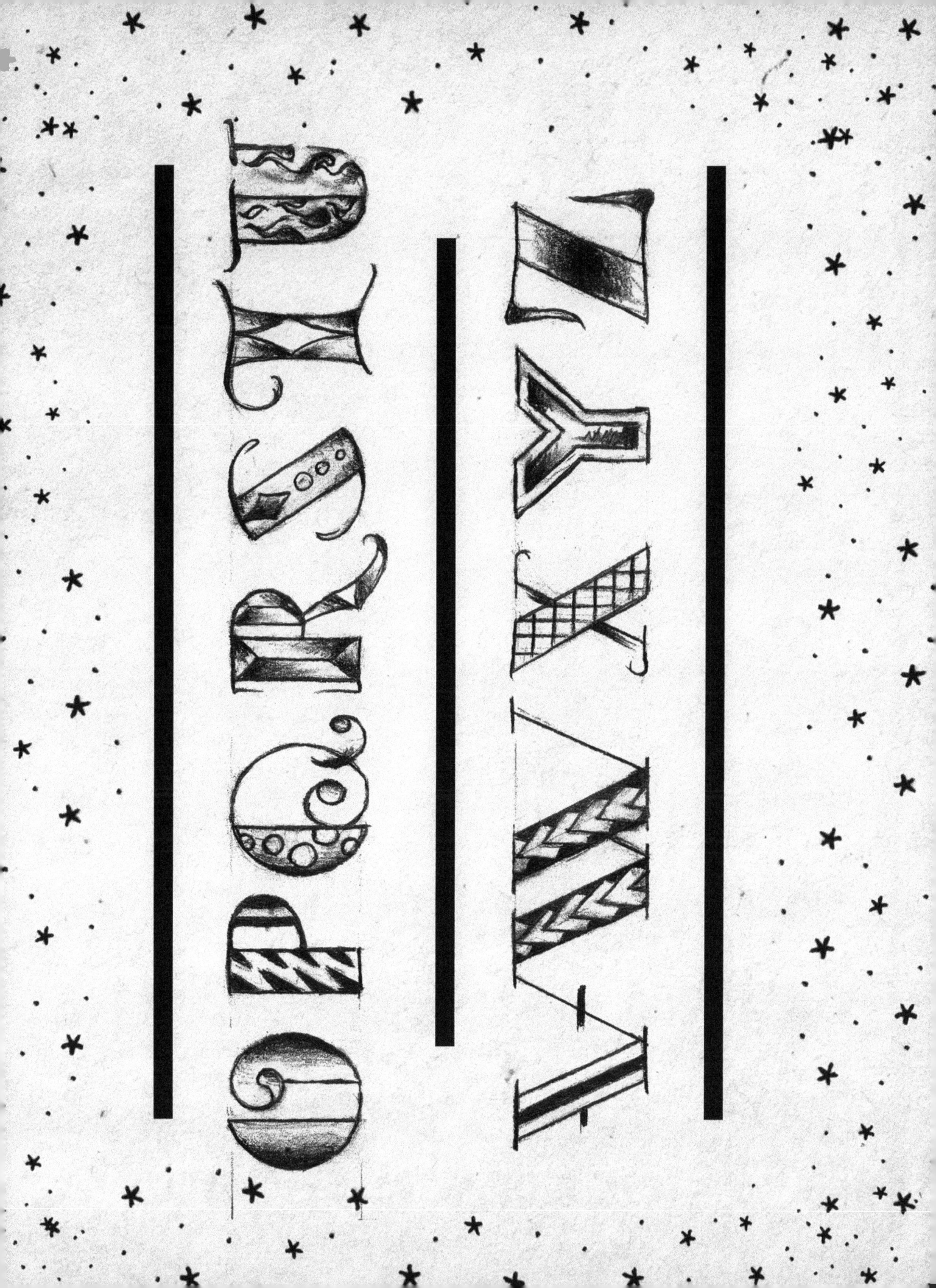

This Too Shall Pass

This Too Shall Pass

This Too Shall Pass

This Too Shall Pass

Don't Tread On Me

Don't Tread On Me

Don't Tread On Me

Don't Tread On Me

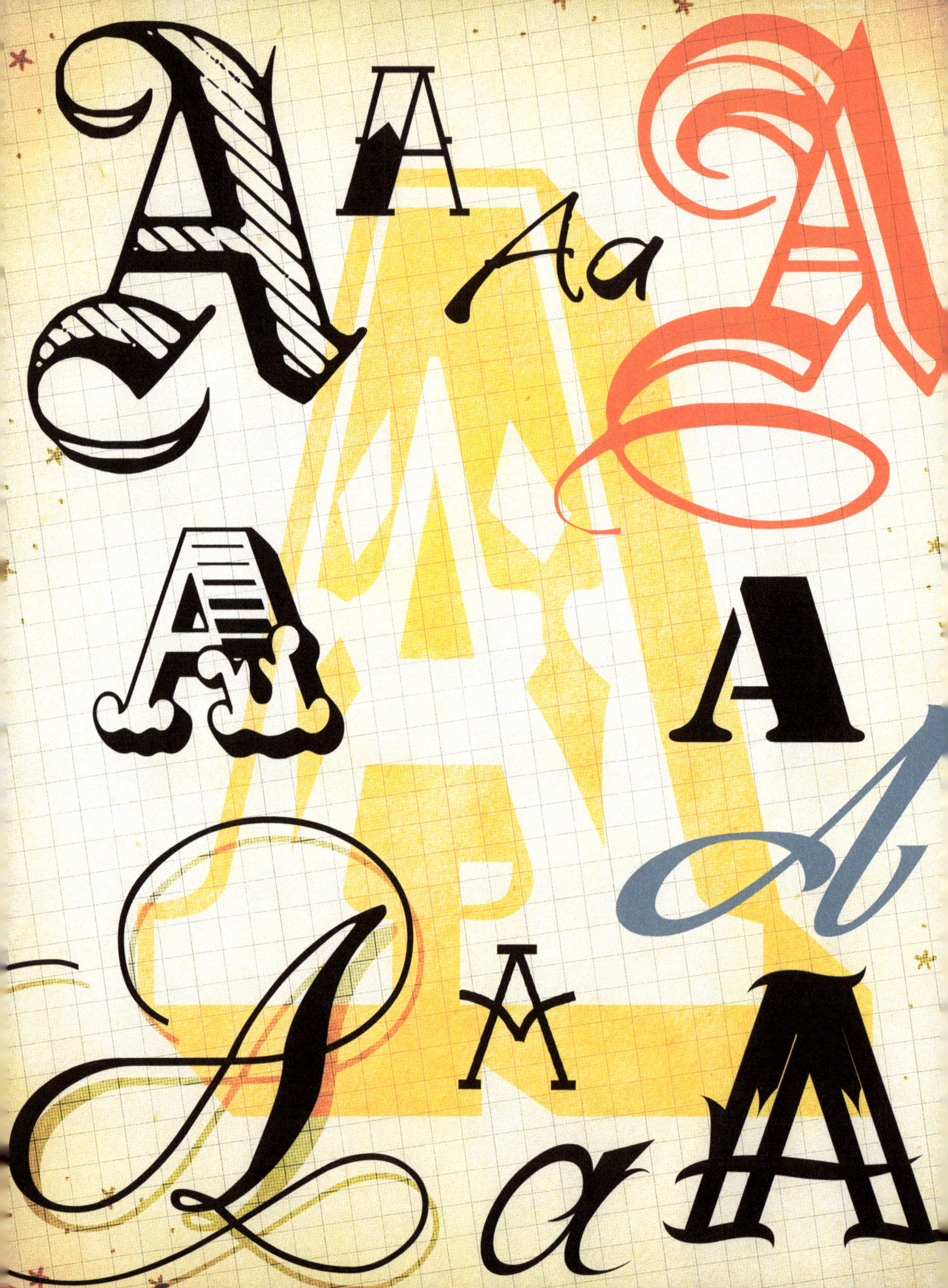

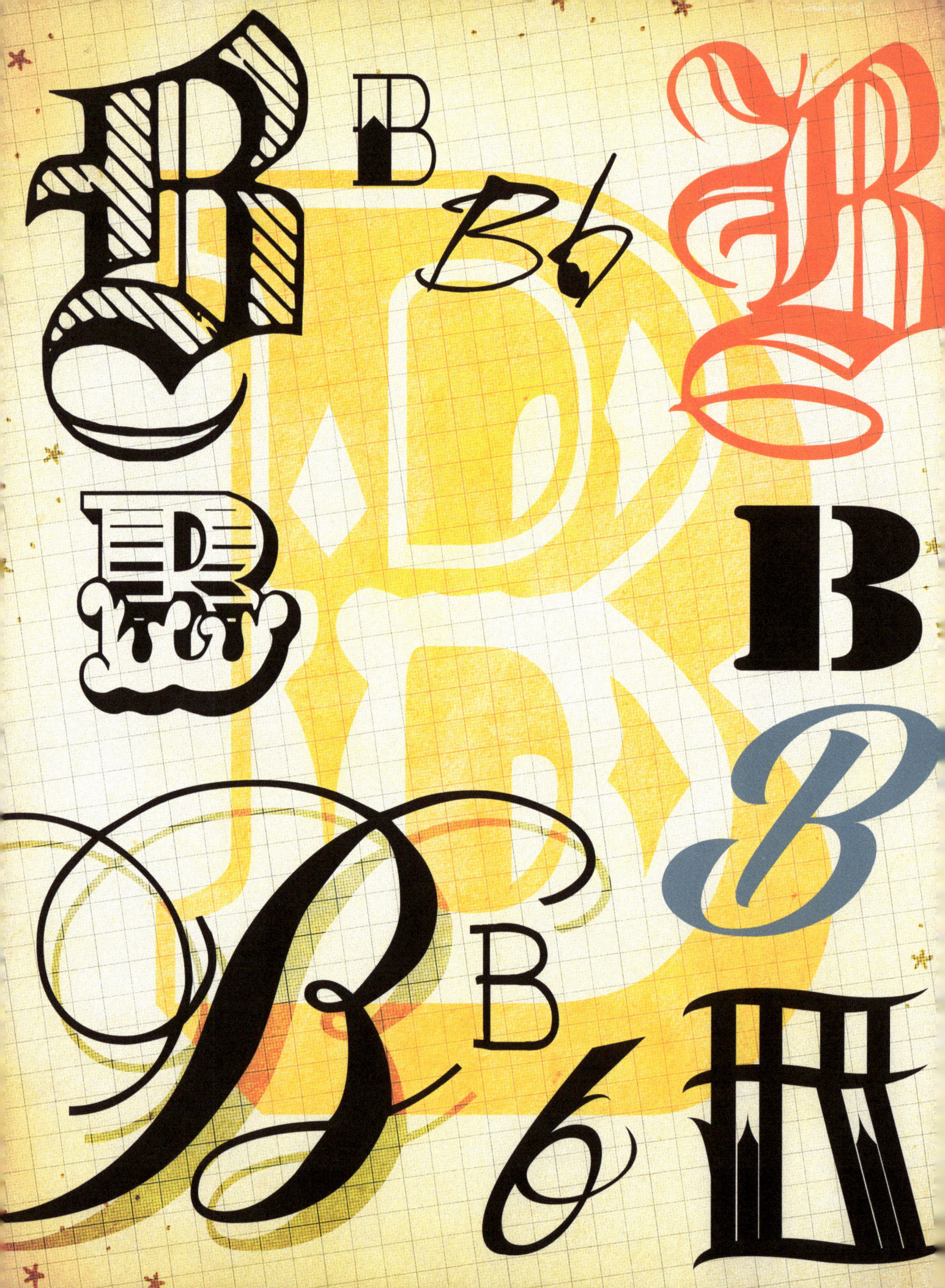

ABCDEFG

HIJKLMN

OPQRST

UVWXYZ

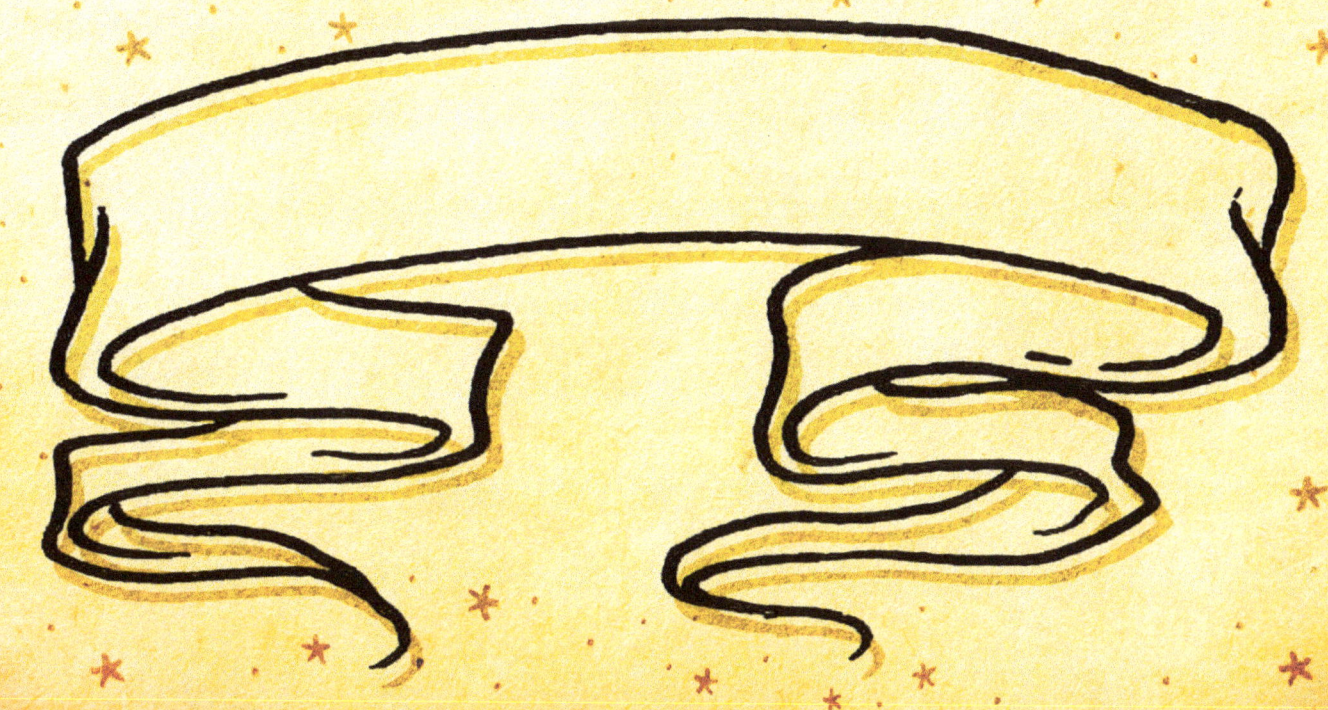

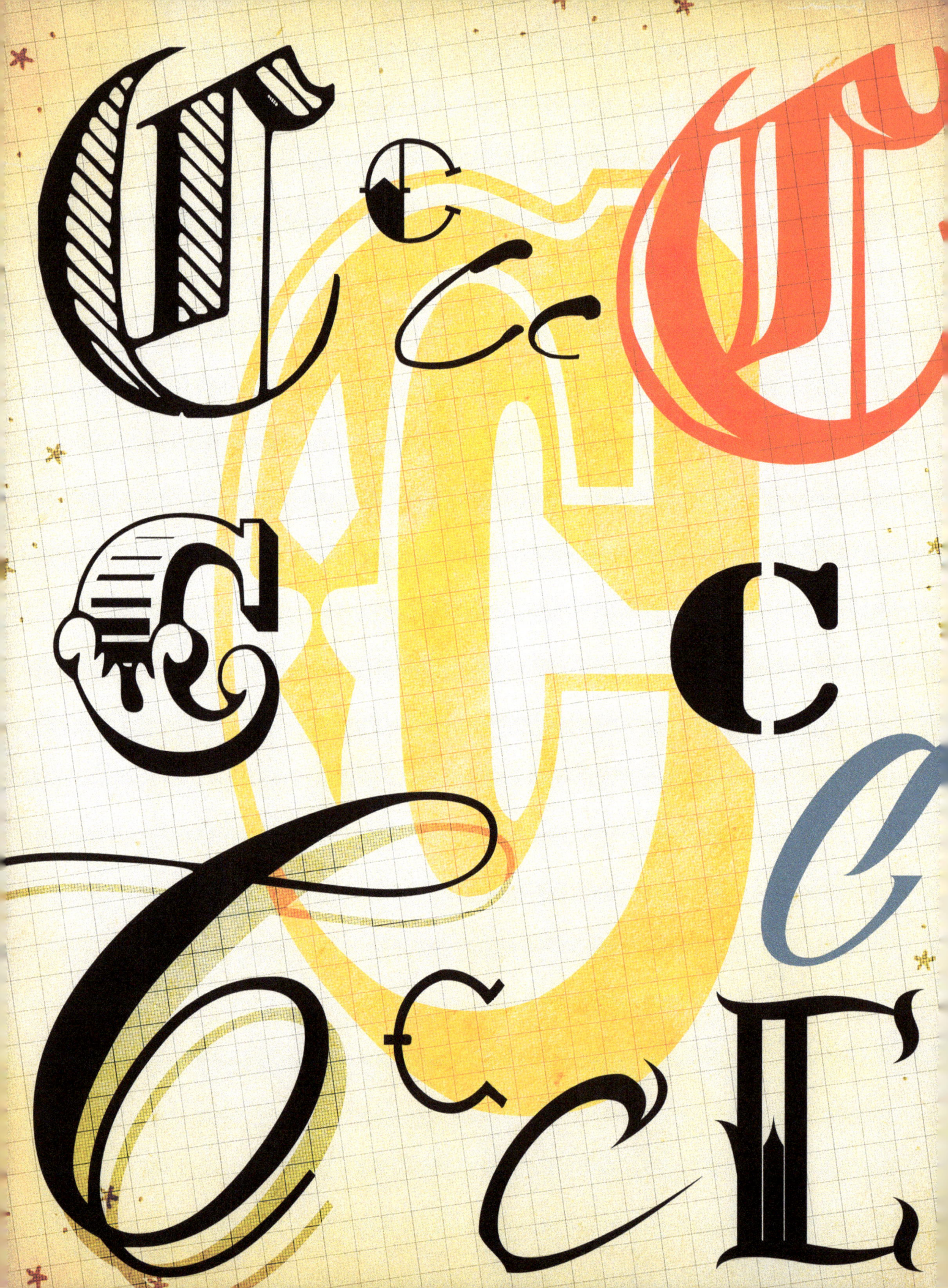

A B C D E F G
H I J K L M N
O P Q R S T U
V W X Y Z

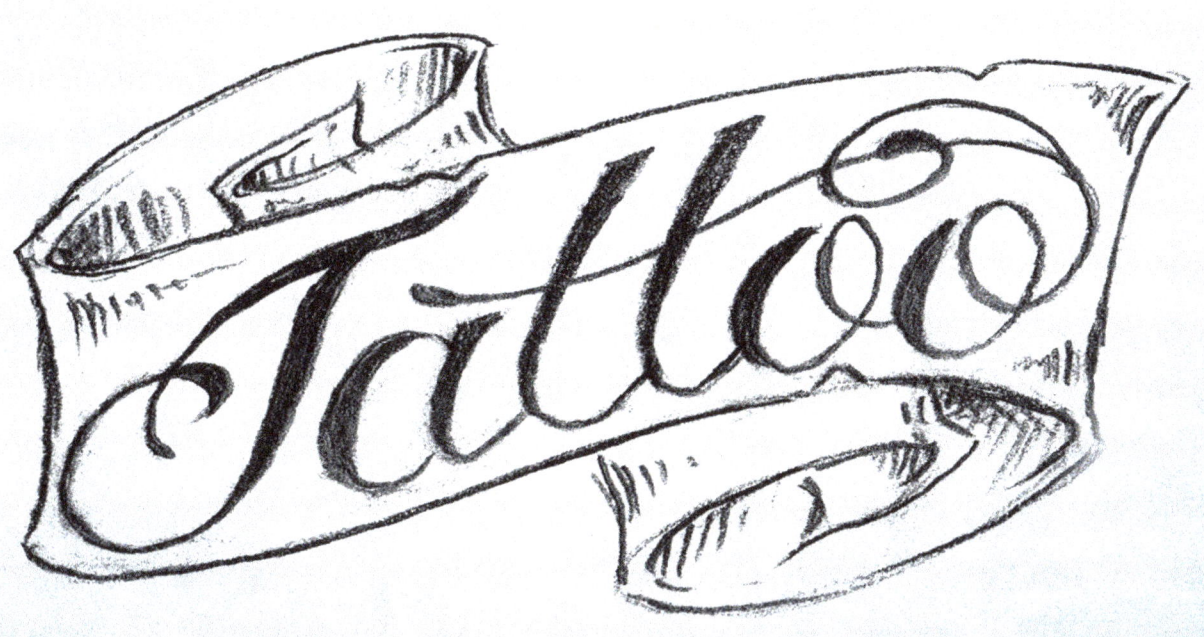

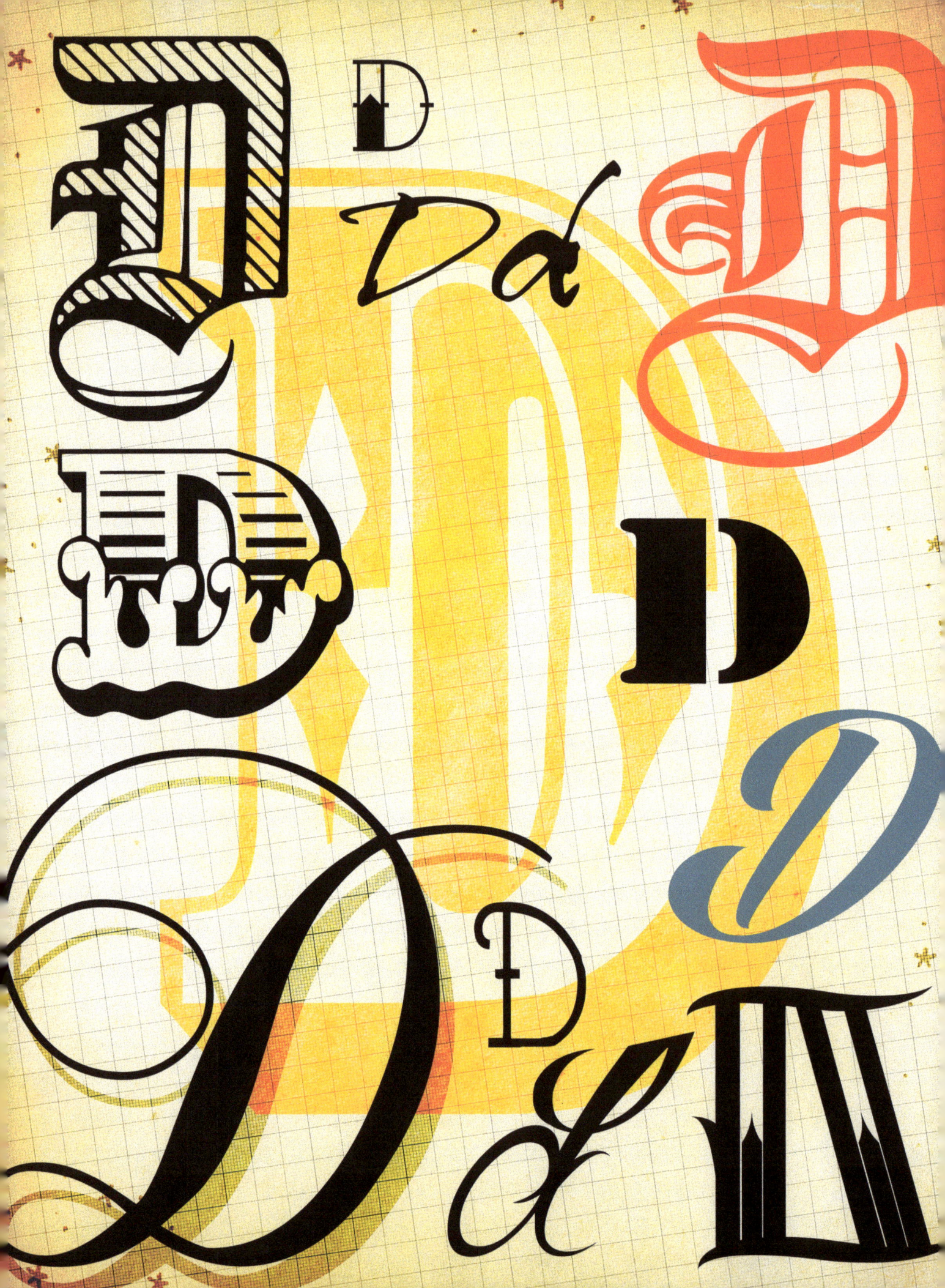

Strength

STRENGTH

Strength

Strength

Strength

Strength

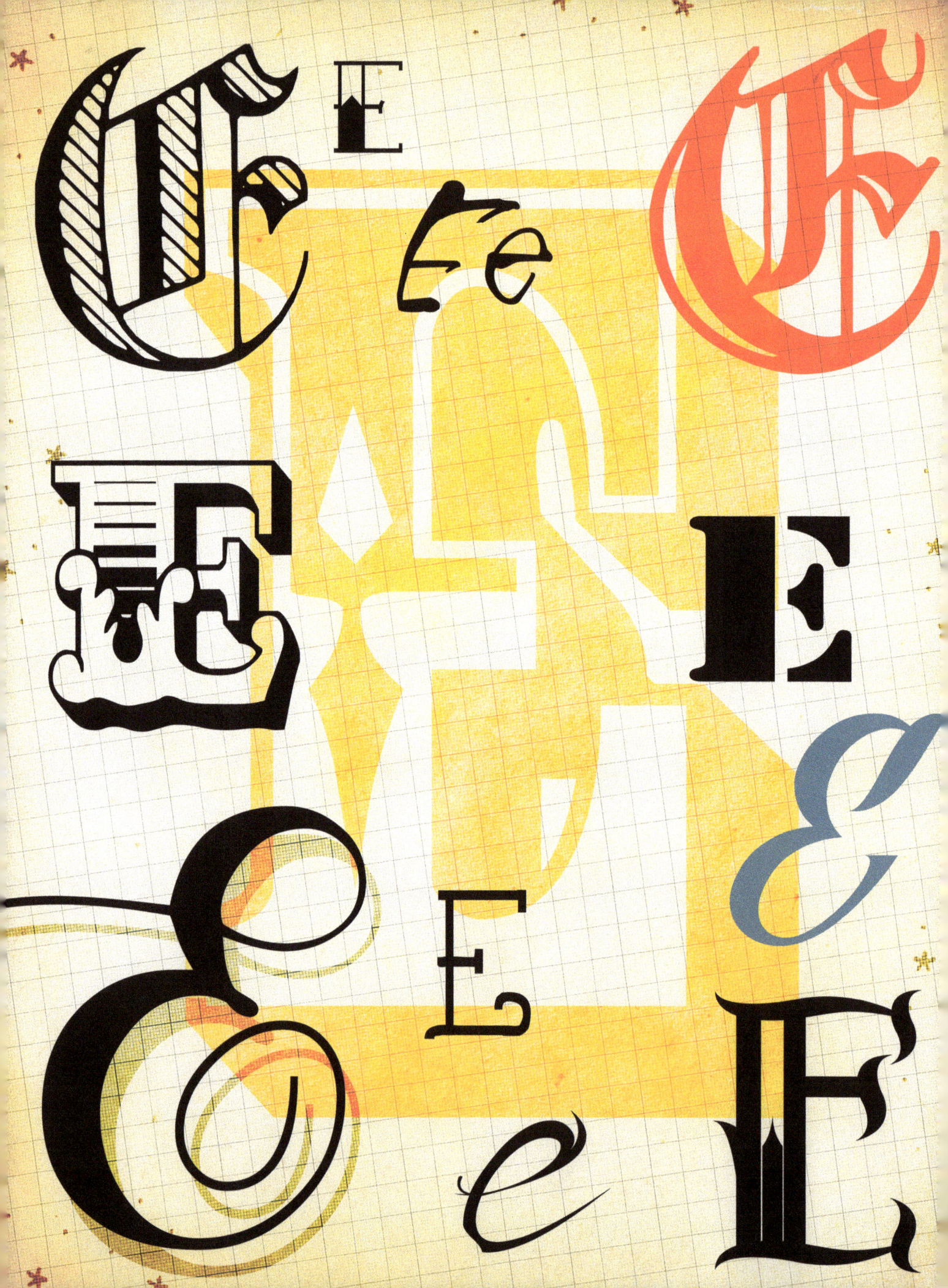

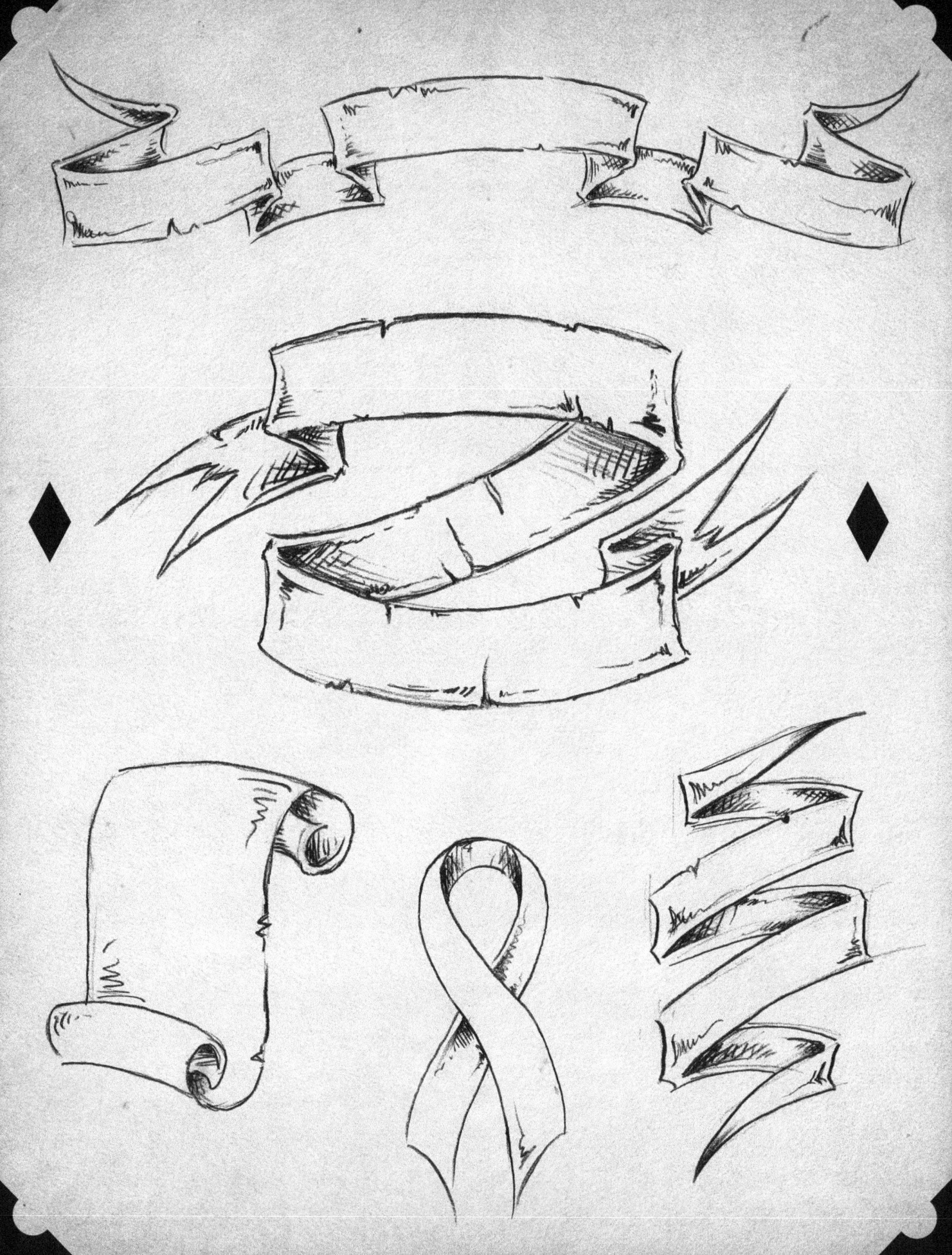

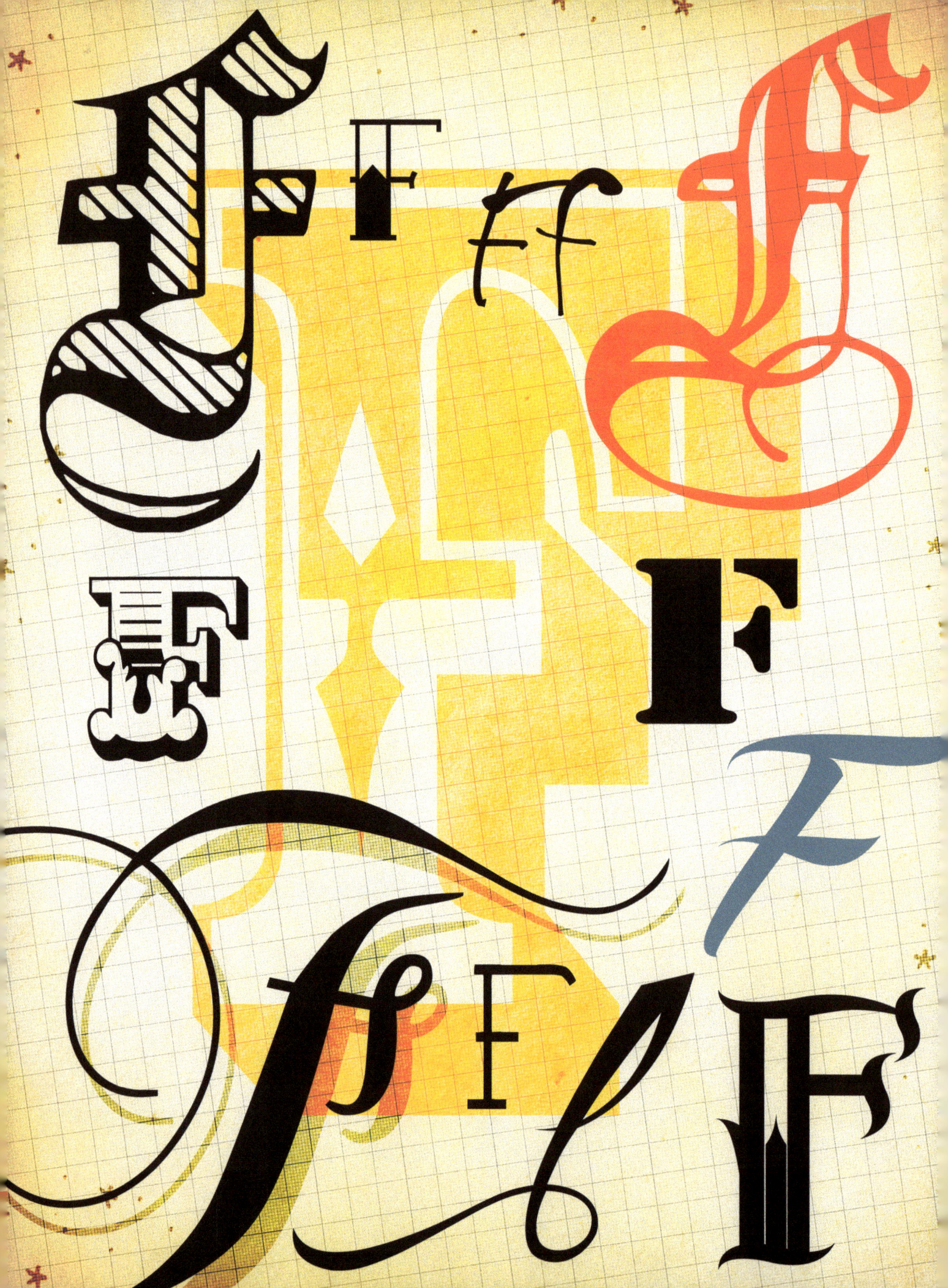

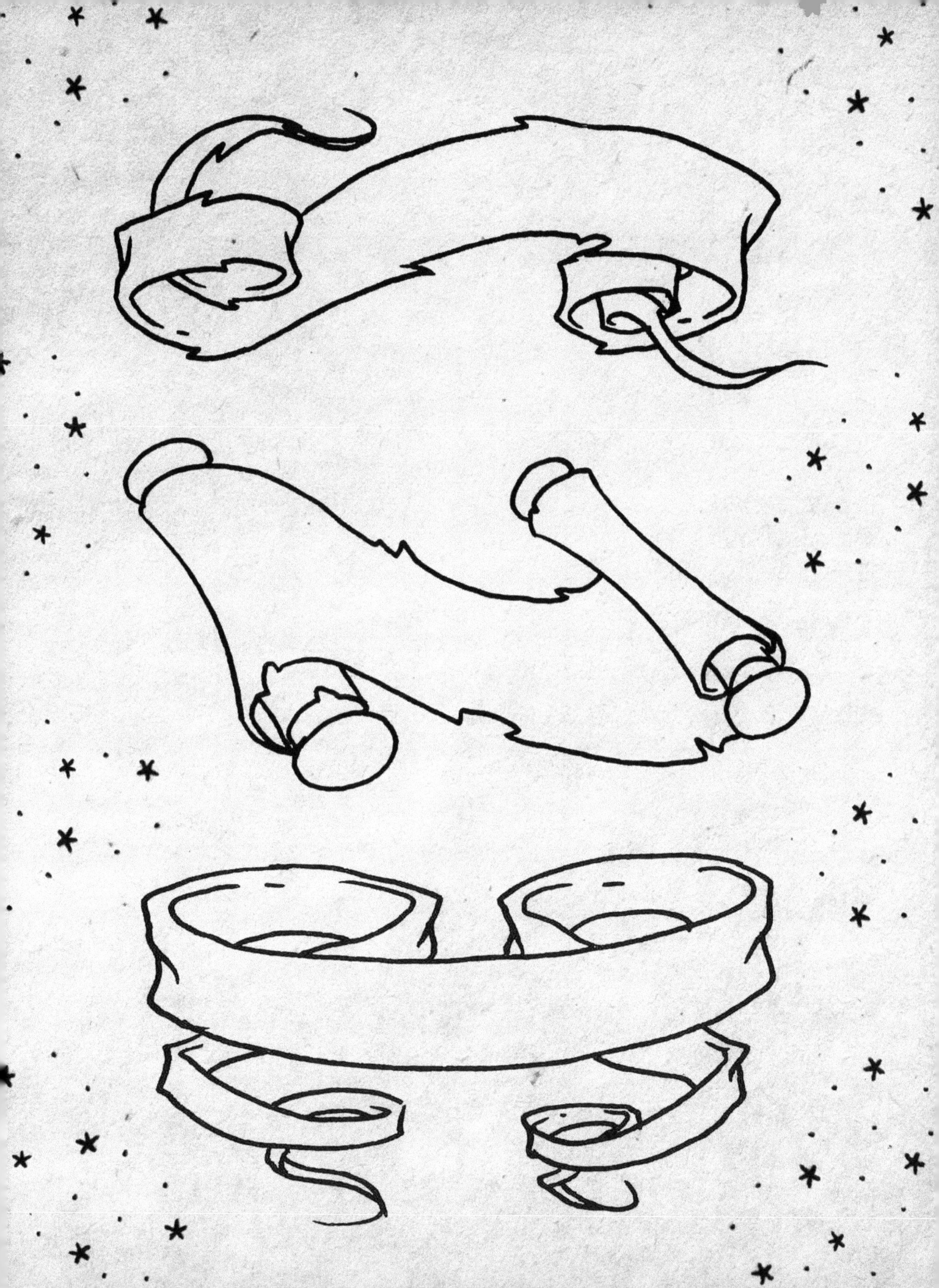

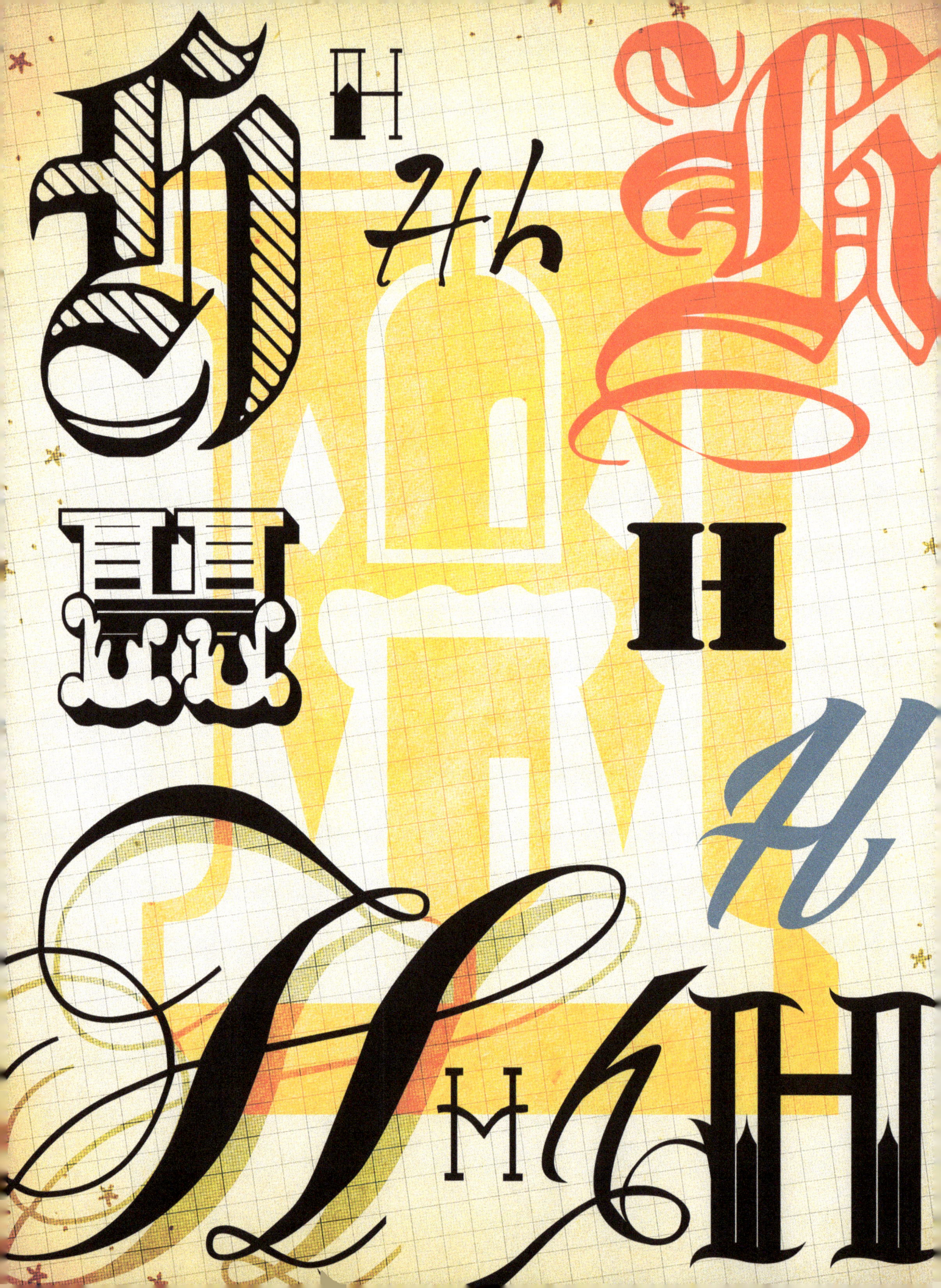

福 Happiness

愛 Love

平 Peace

孚 Truth

忠 Loyalty

和 Harmony

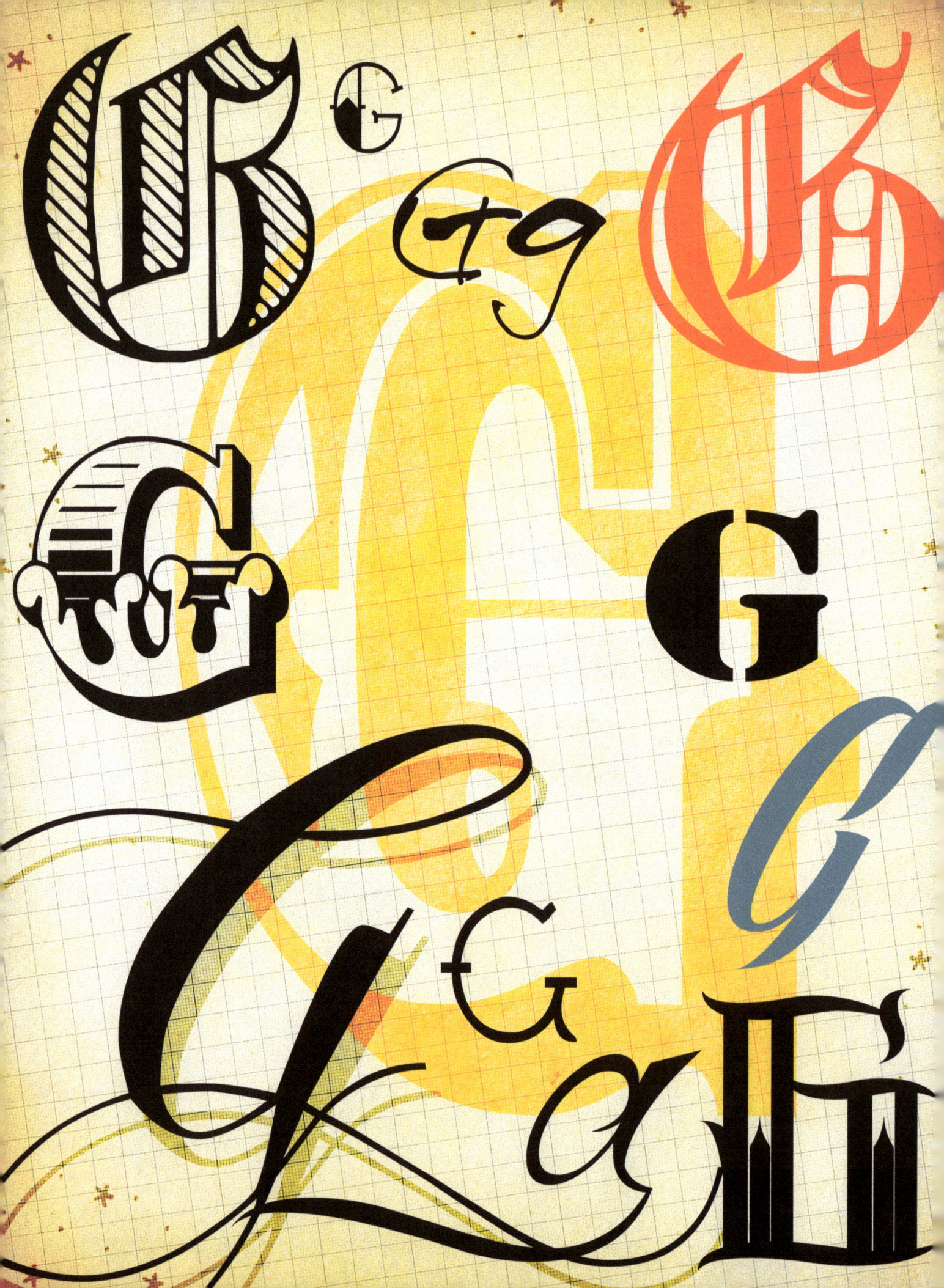

Nothing Is Forever
Nothing Is Forever
Nothing Is Forever
Nothing Is Forever

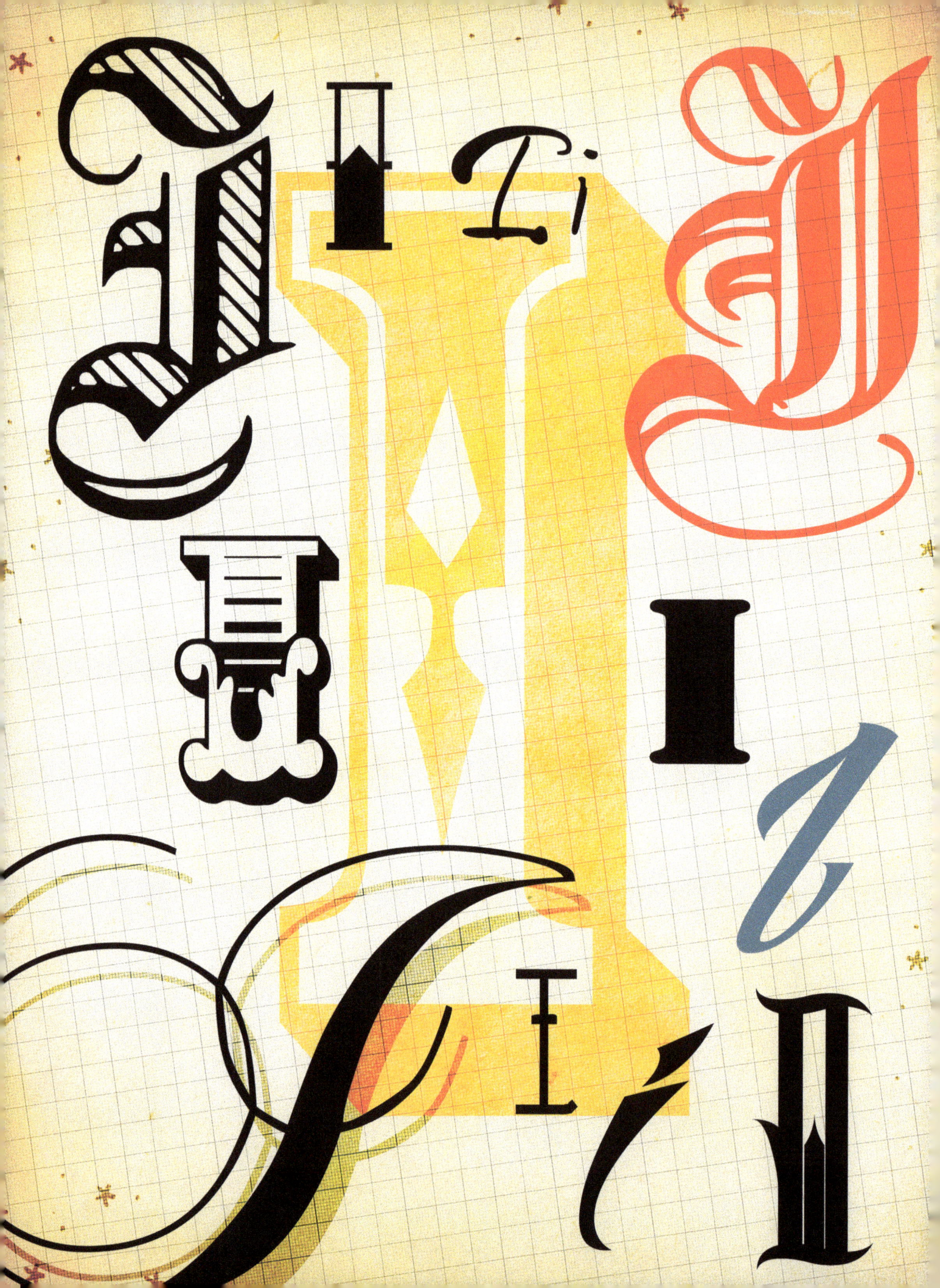

ABCDEFGH
IJKLMNOPQ
RSTUVWXYZ

TATTOO

Faith
Love

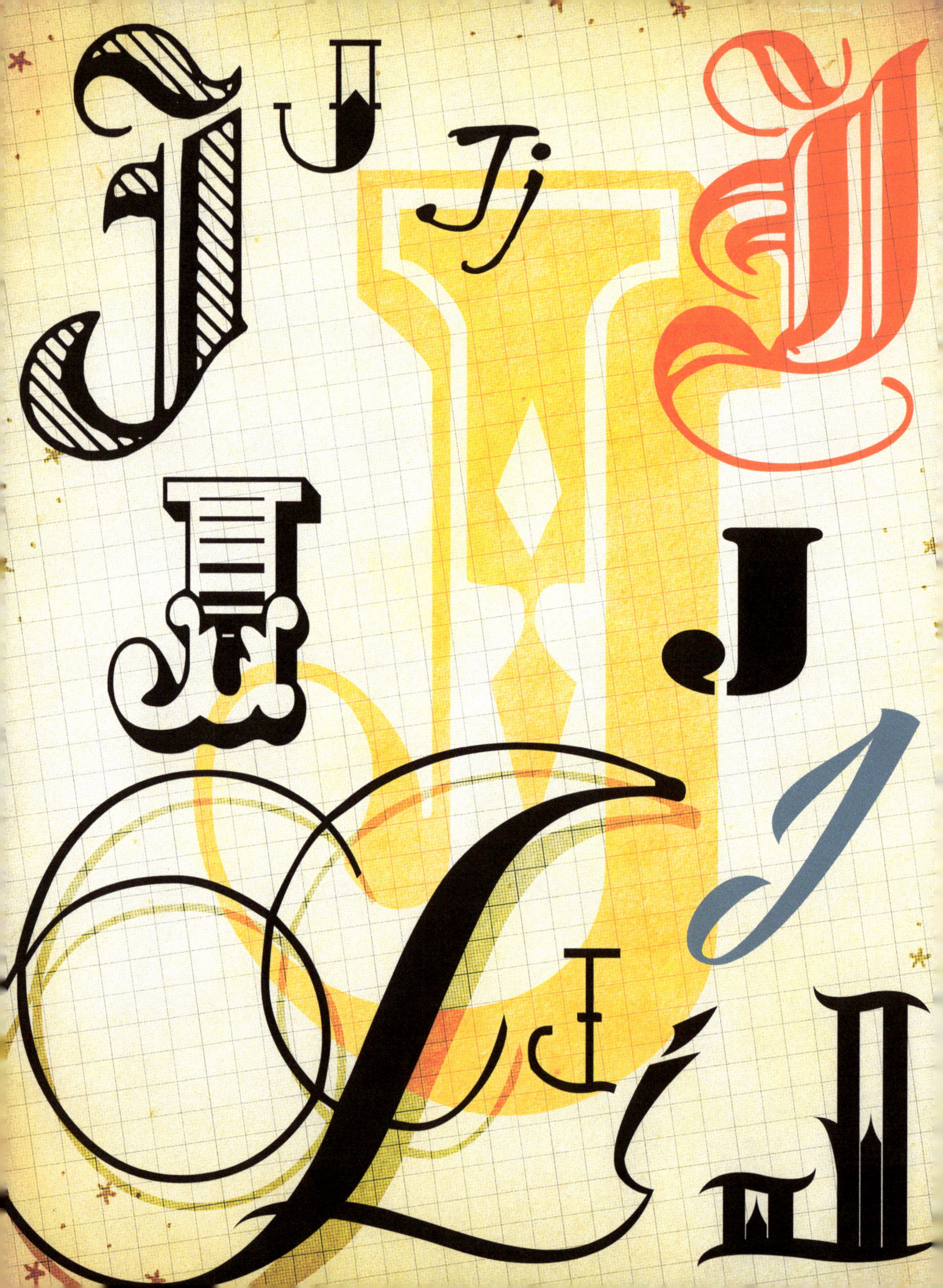

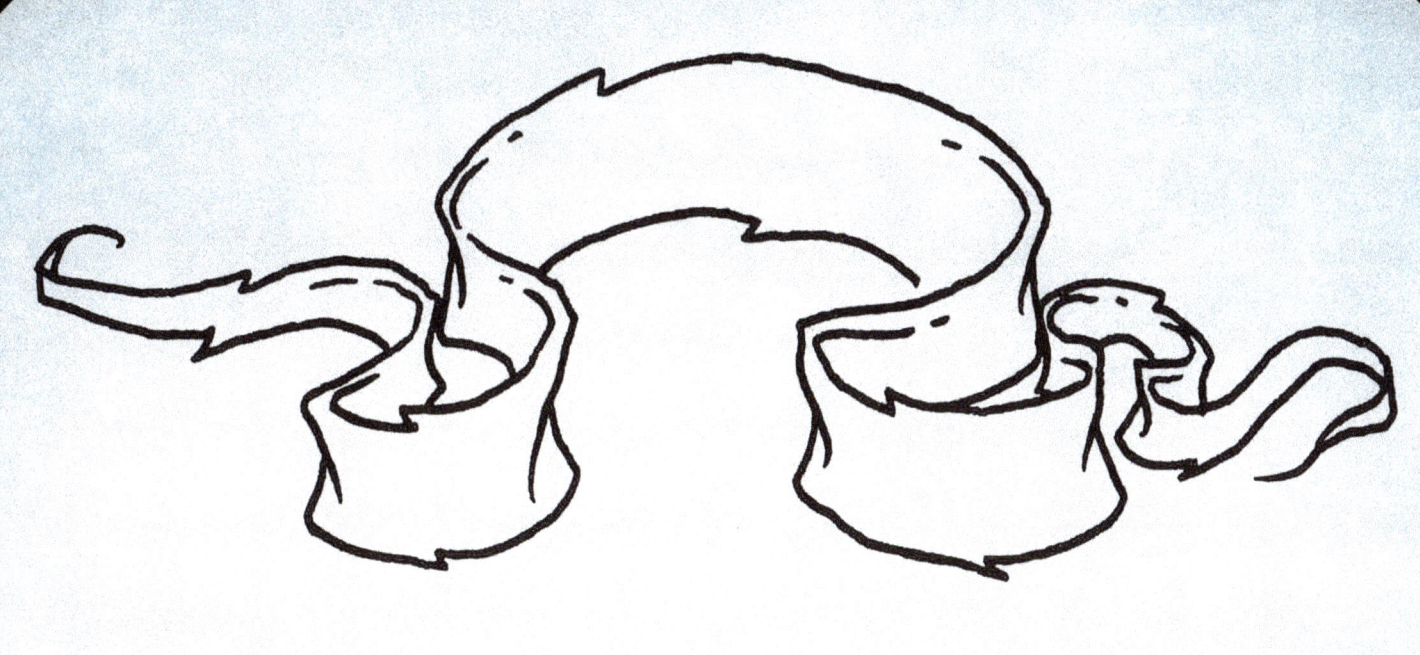

*abcdefgh
ijklmno
pqrst
uvwxyz*

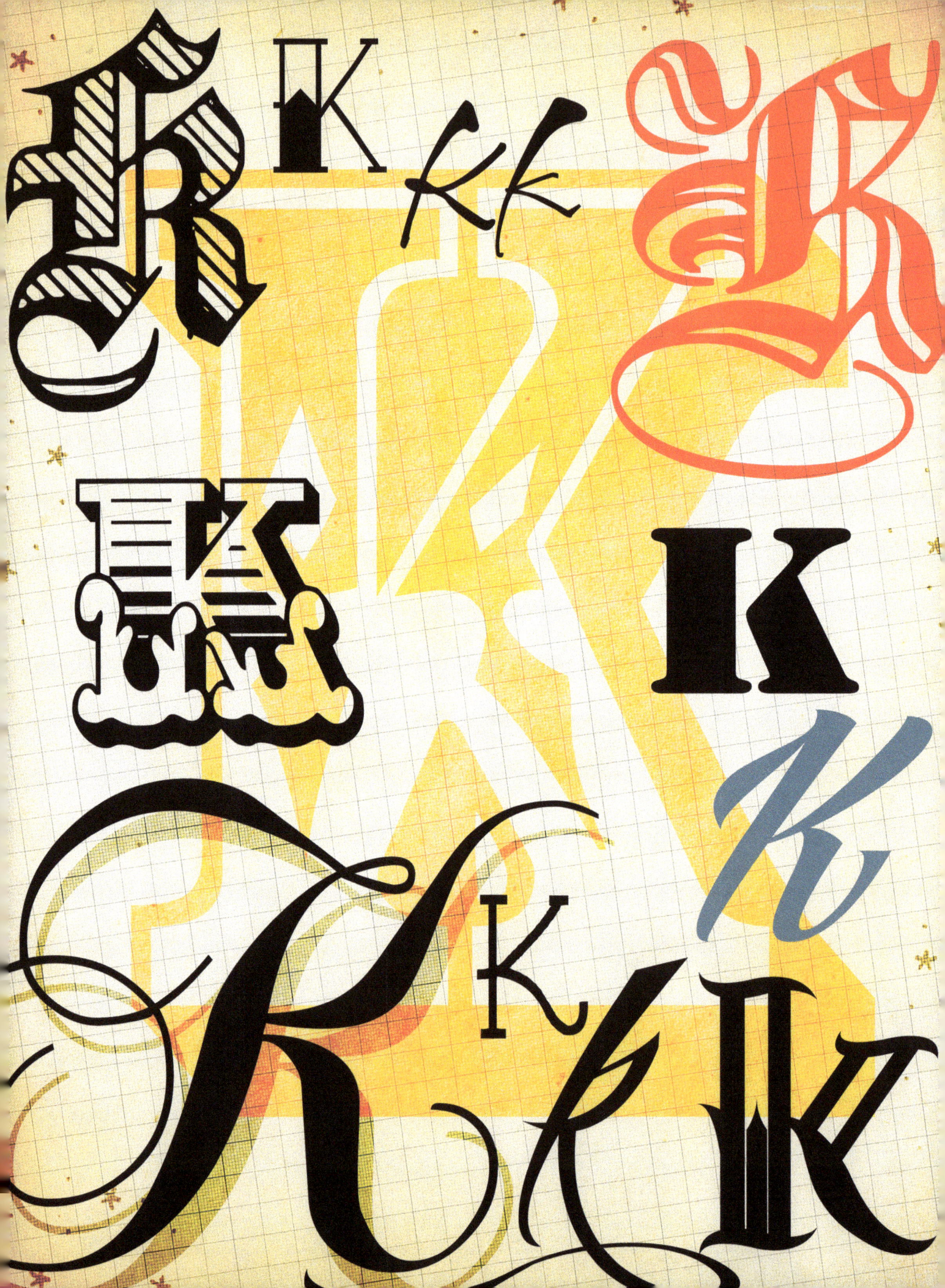

Evil / Evil / Evil

Evil / Evil / Evil

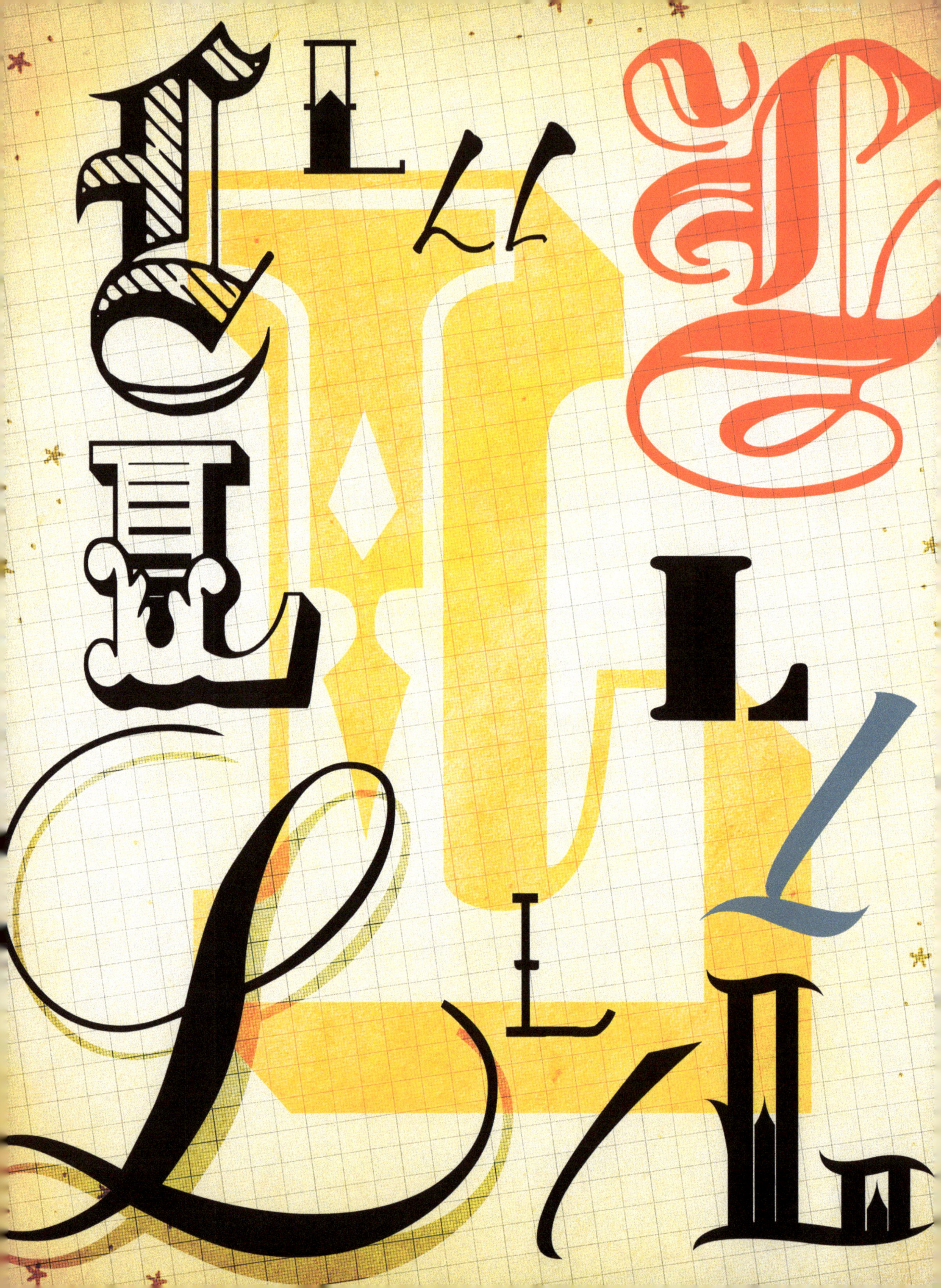

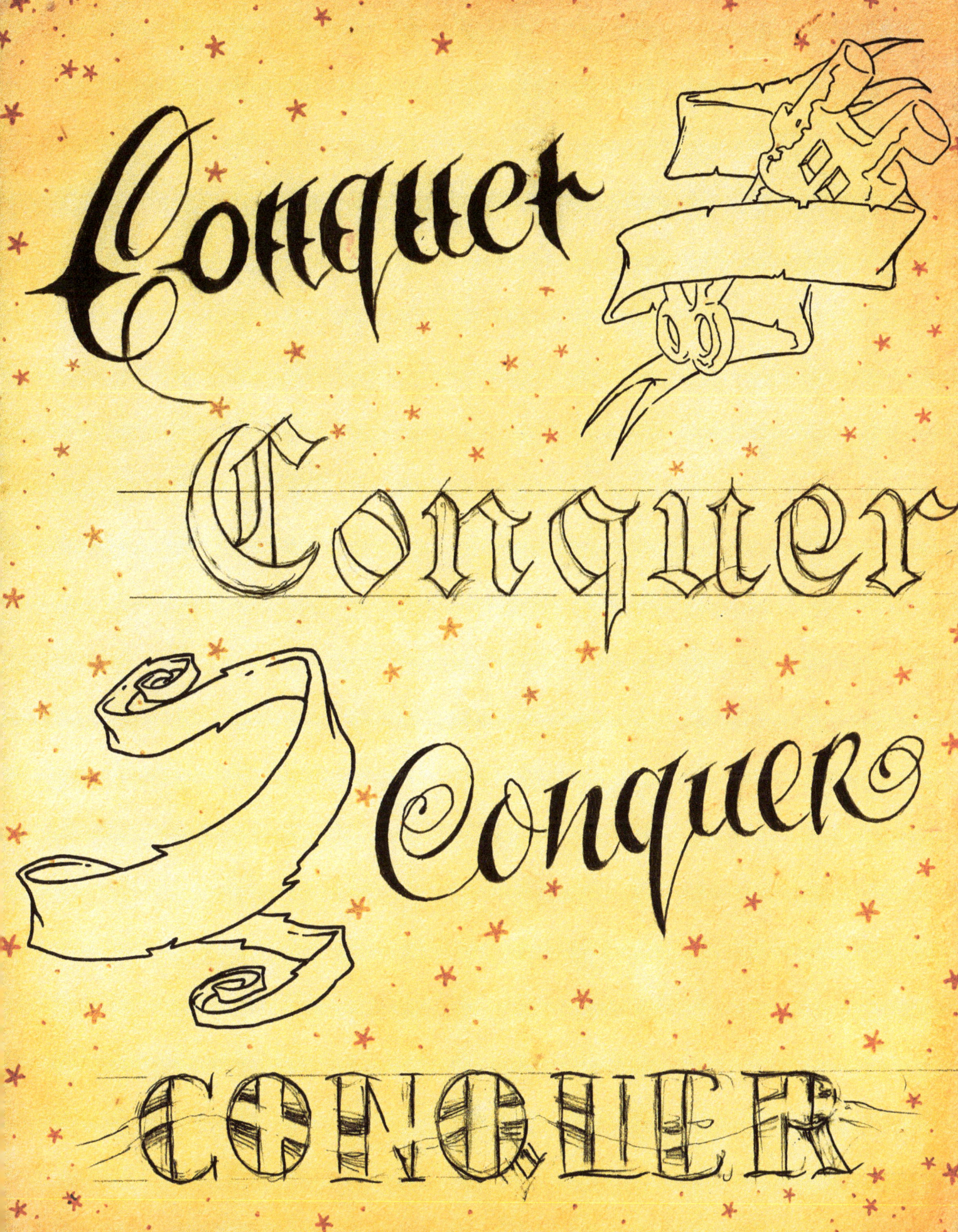

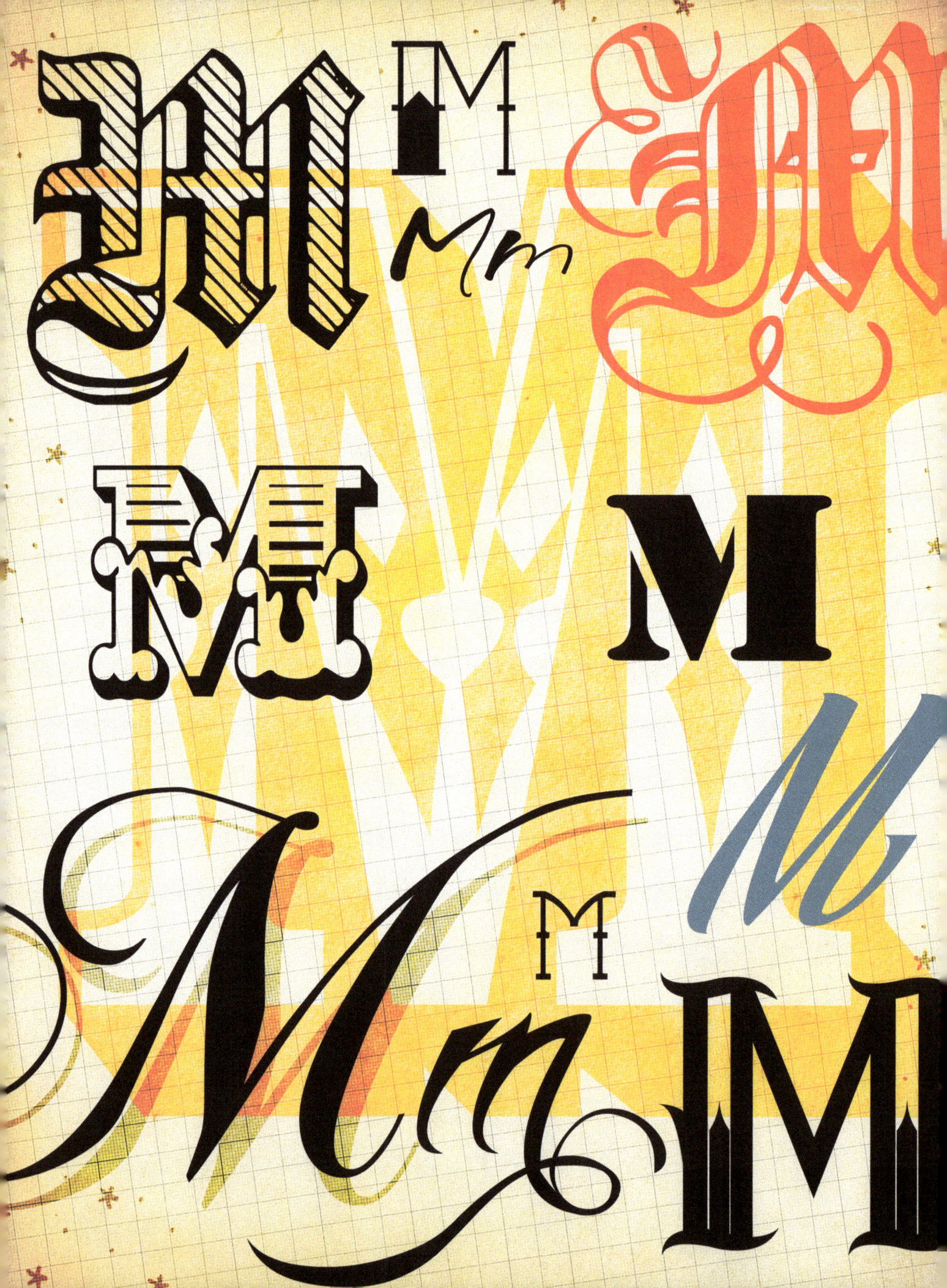

STEAMPUNK

CHINESE

✦ IRISH ✦

ROCKY

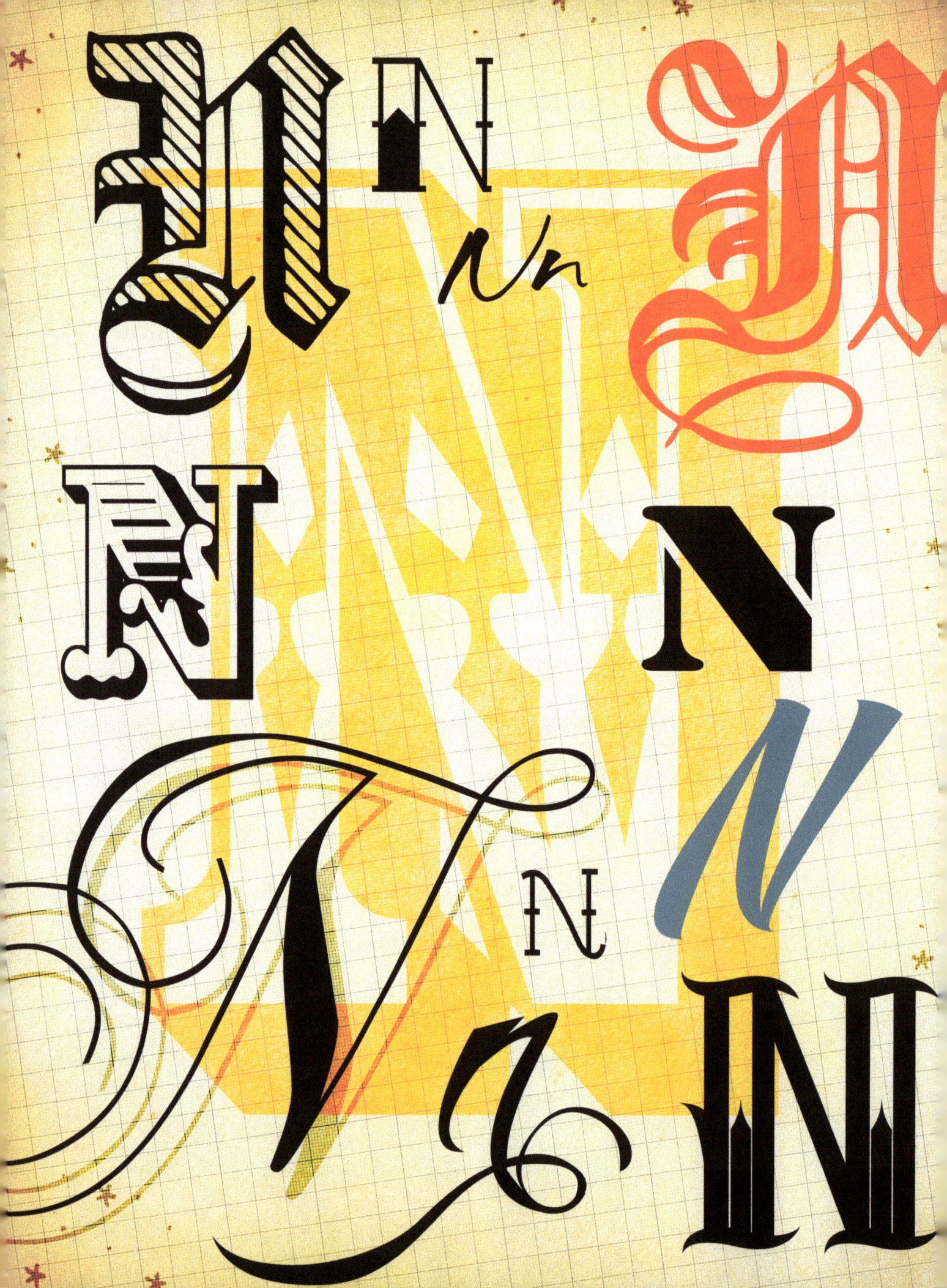

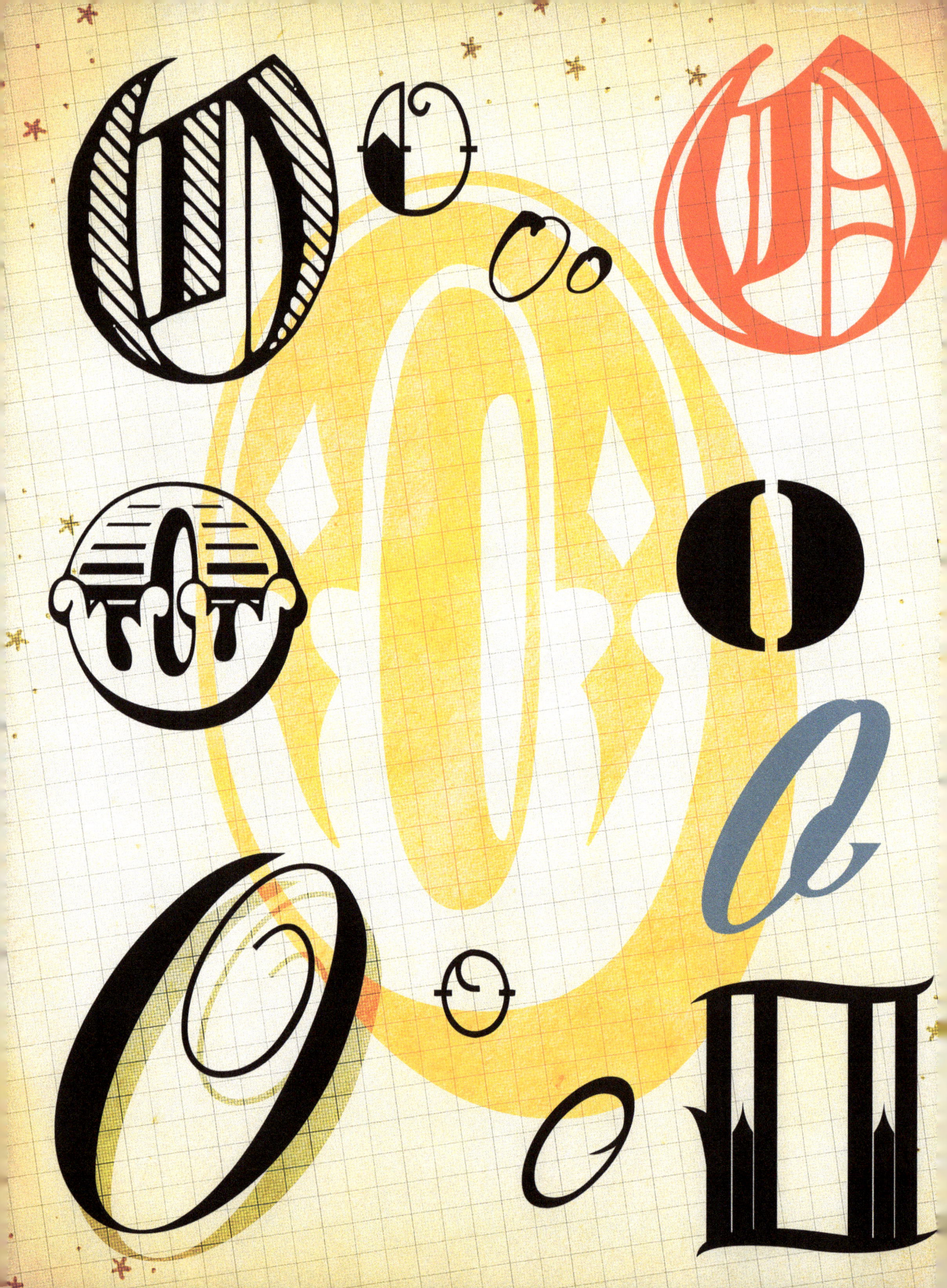

ABCDE
FGHIJK
LMNOPQN
RSTUV
WXYZ

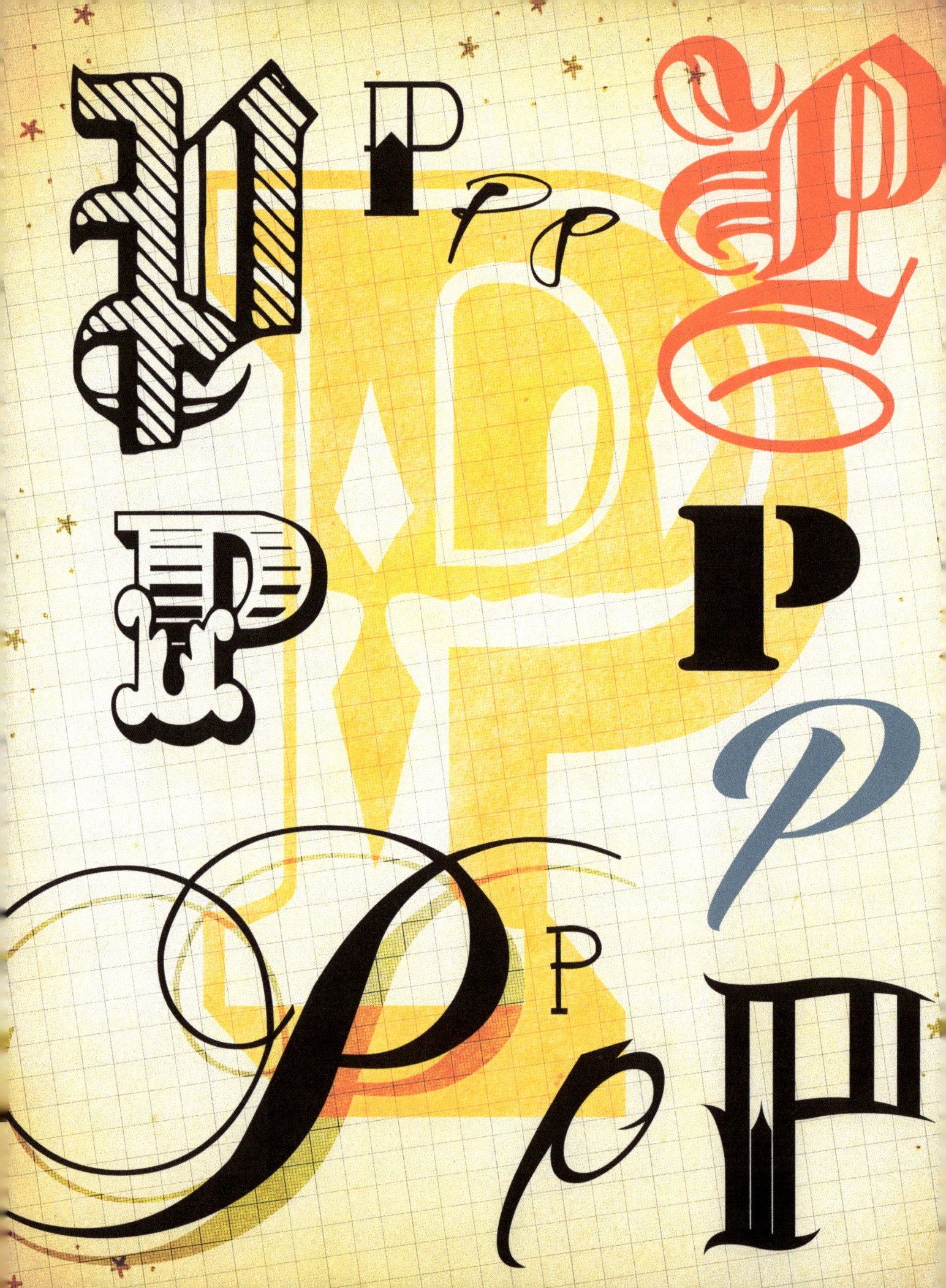

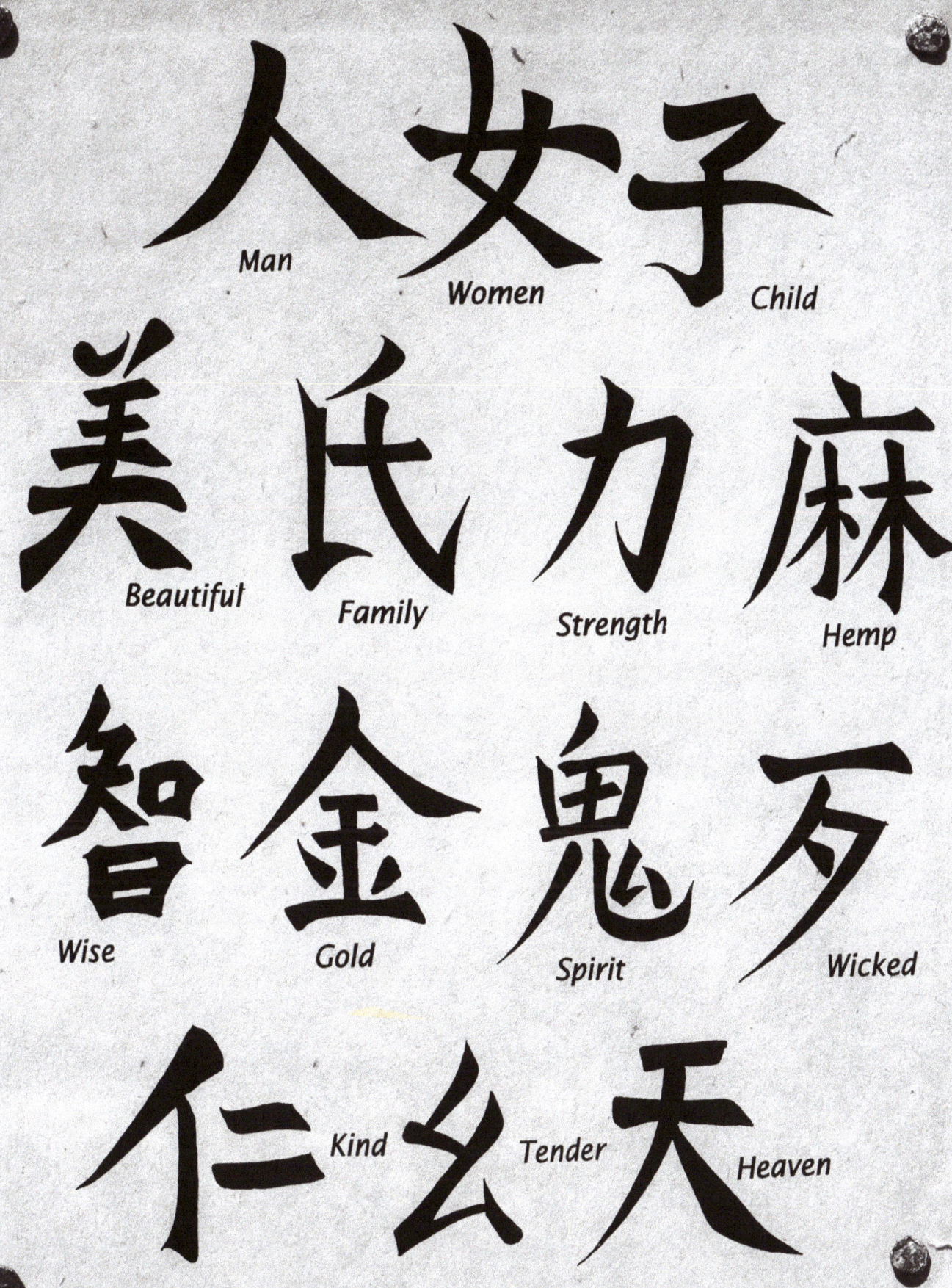

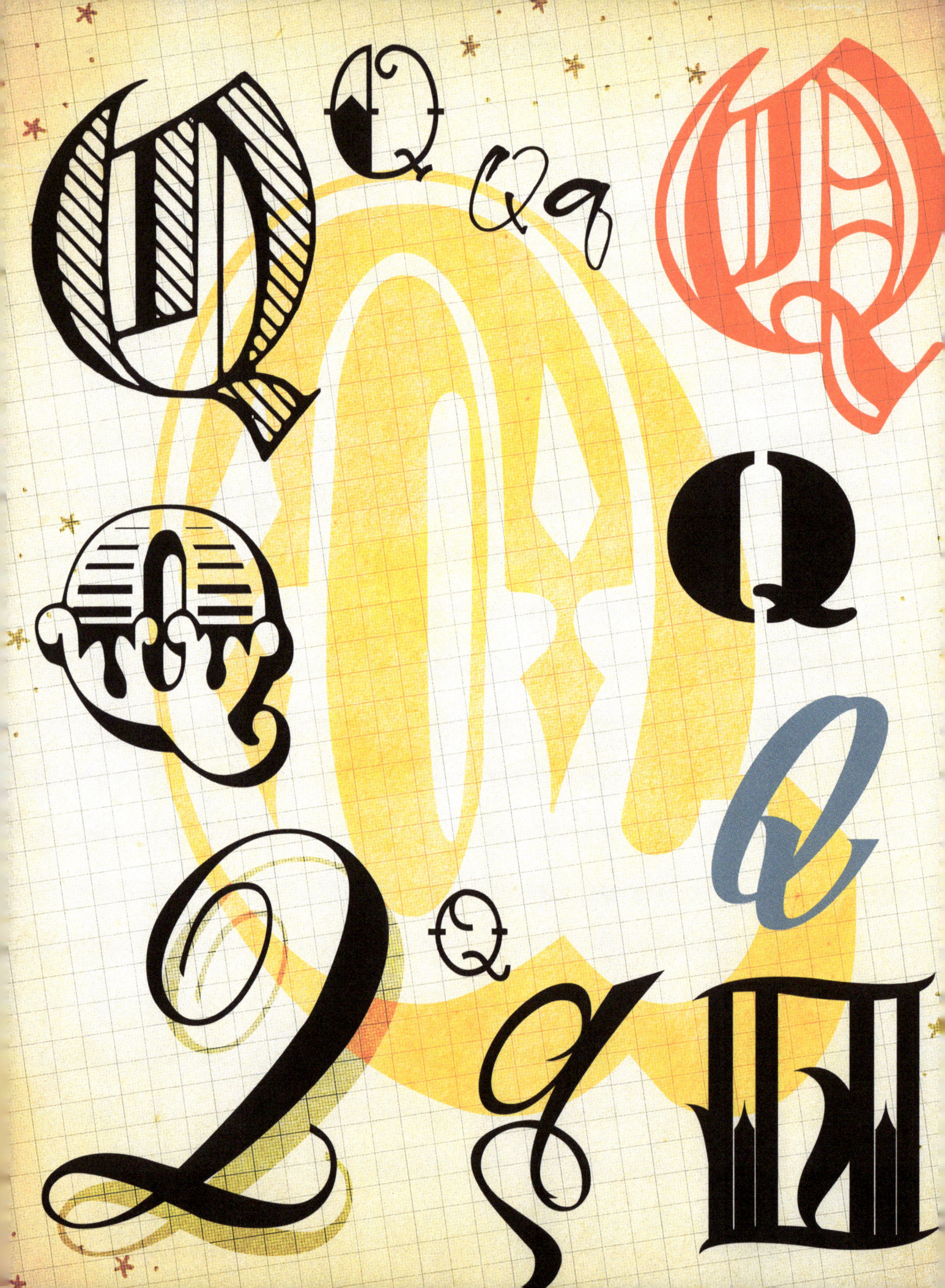

abcdefghijkl mnopqrstu vwxyz

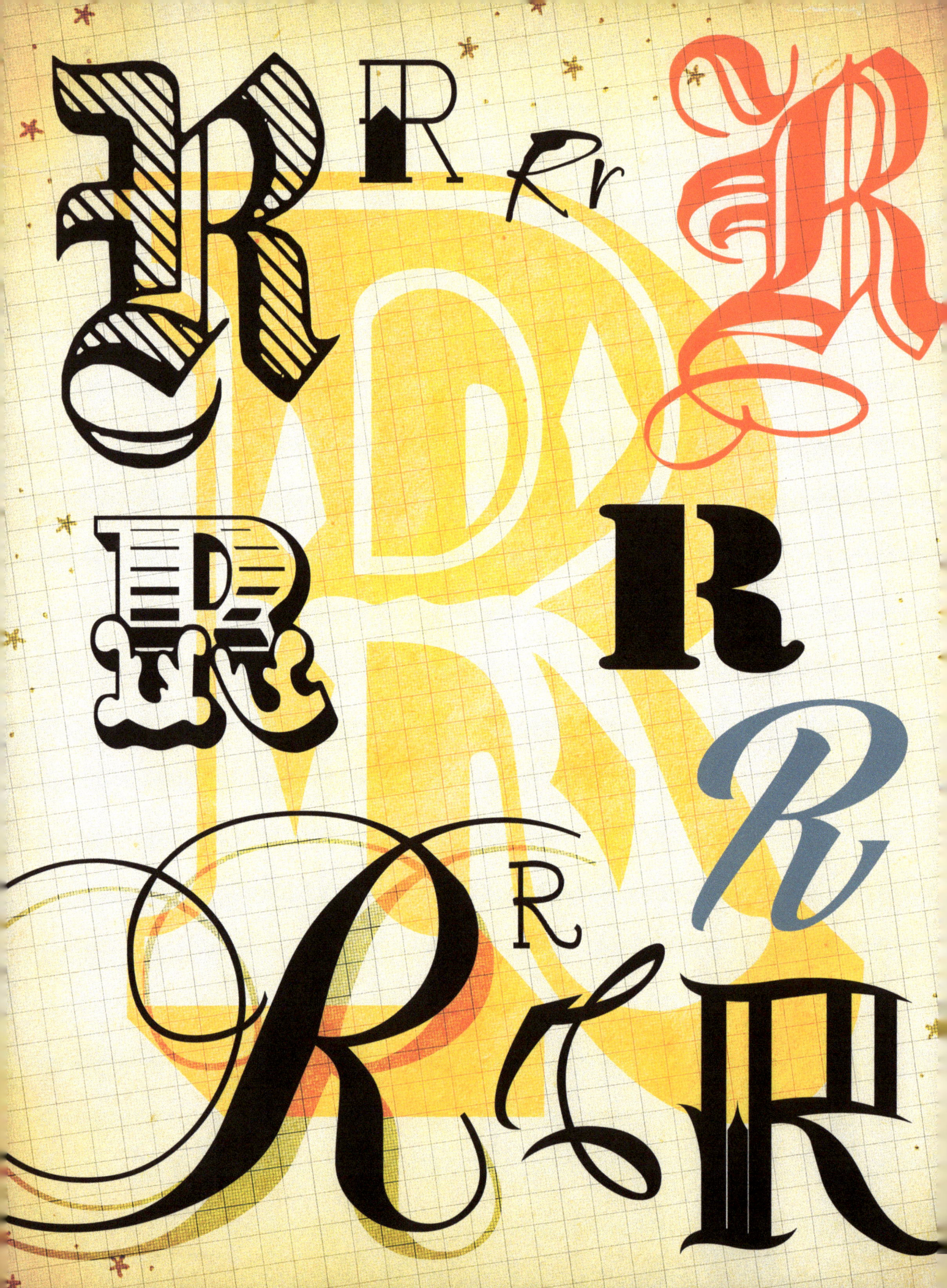

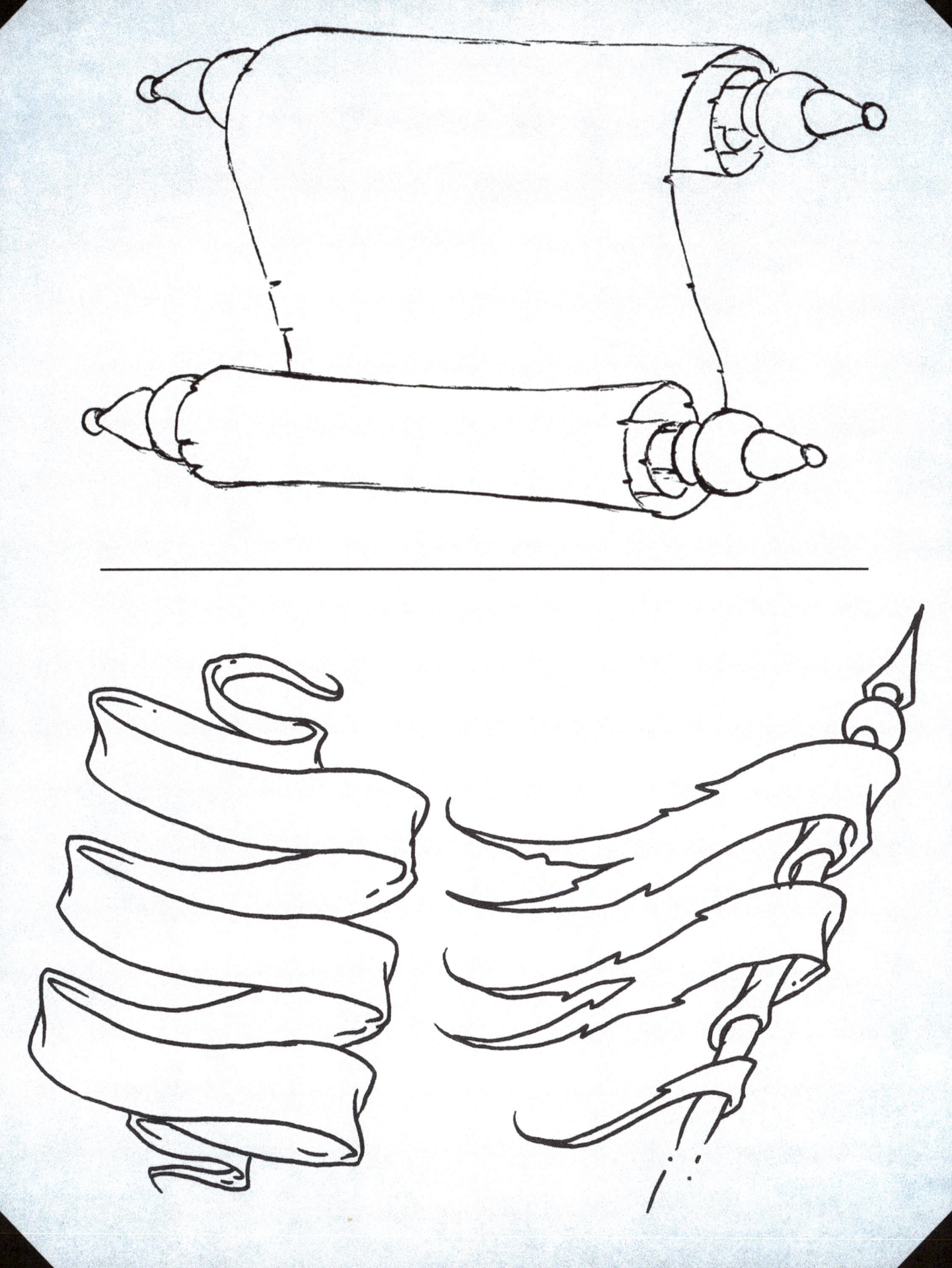

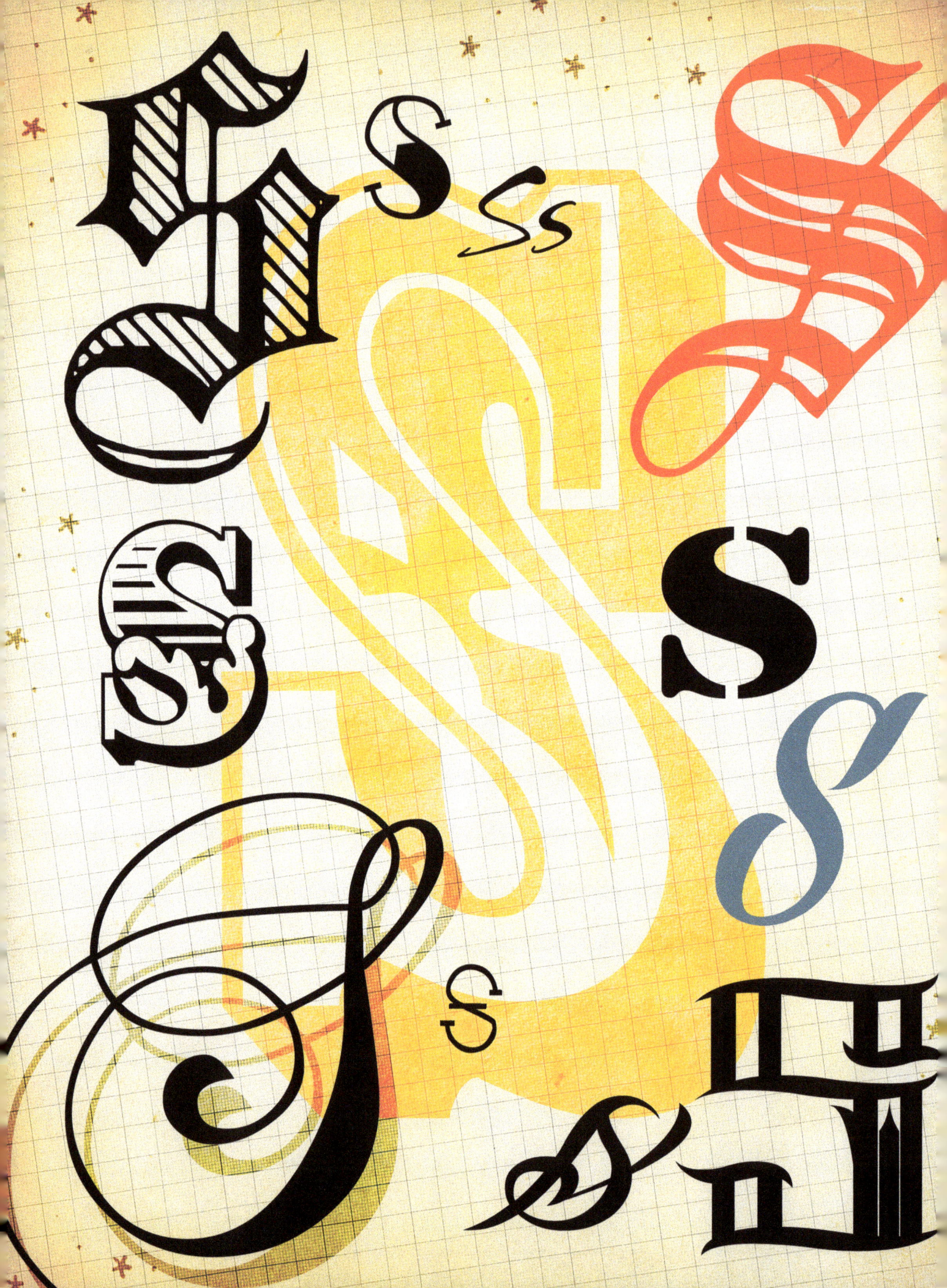

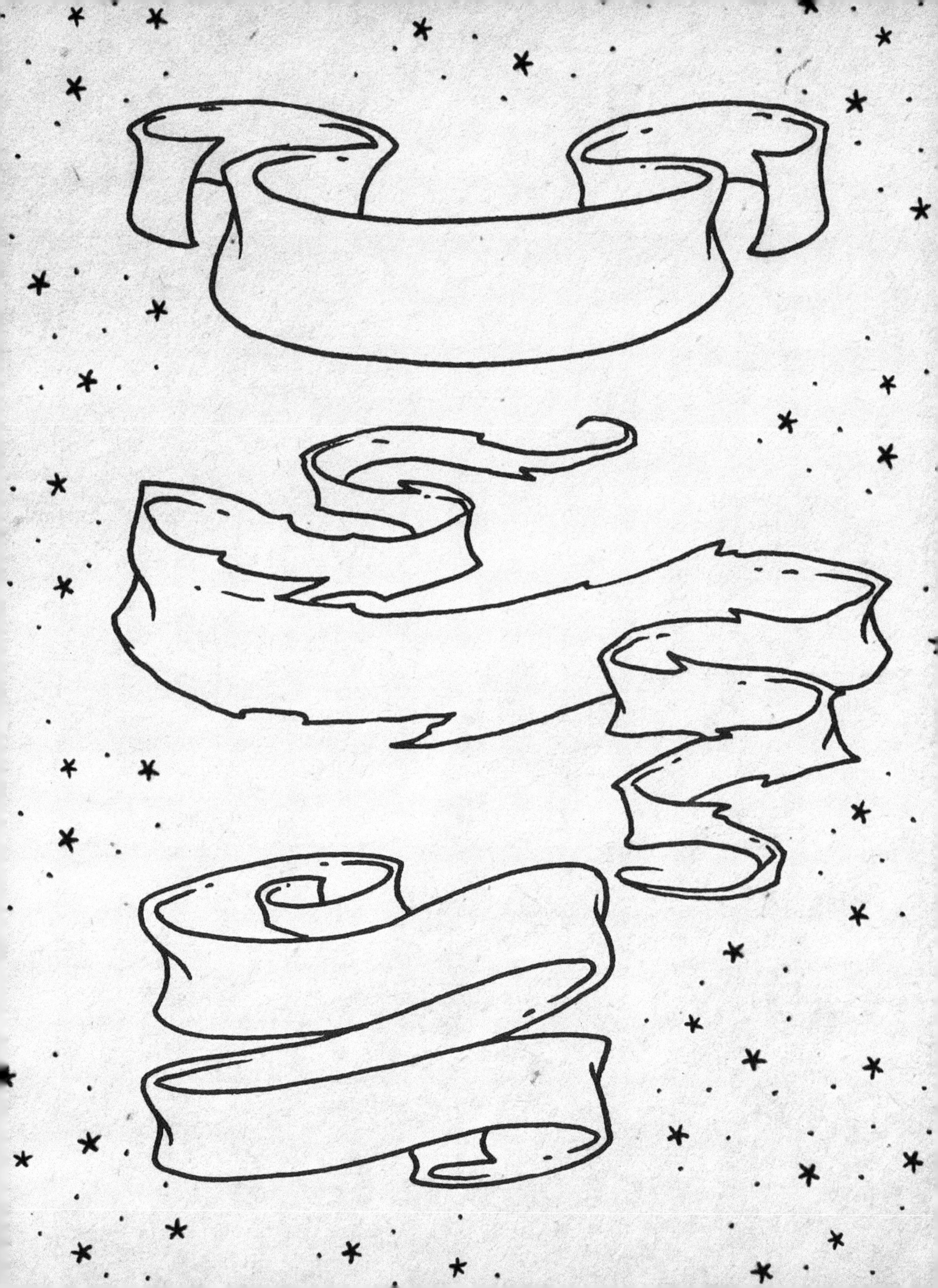

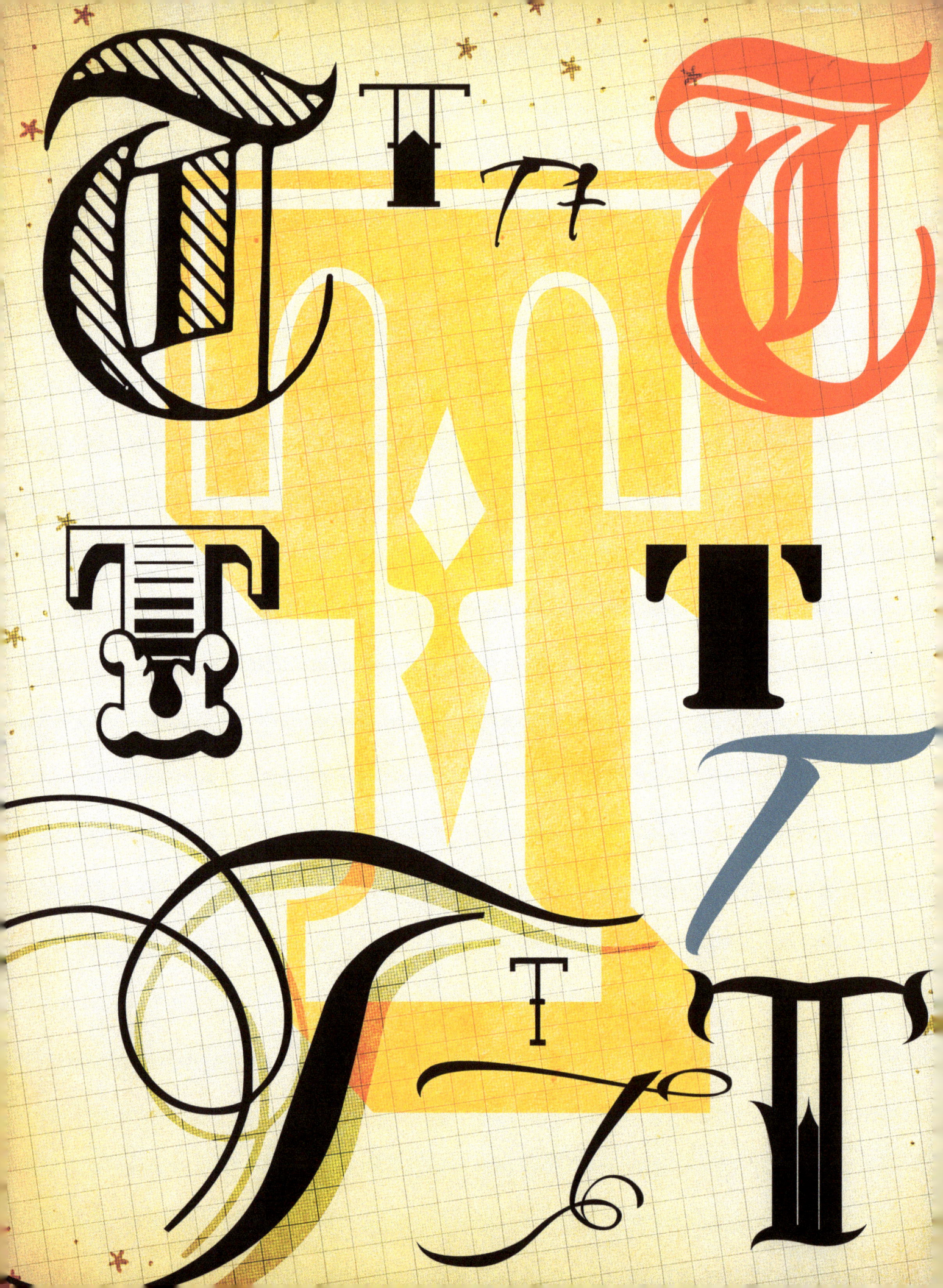

Carpe Diem

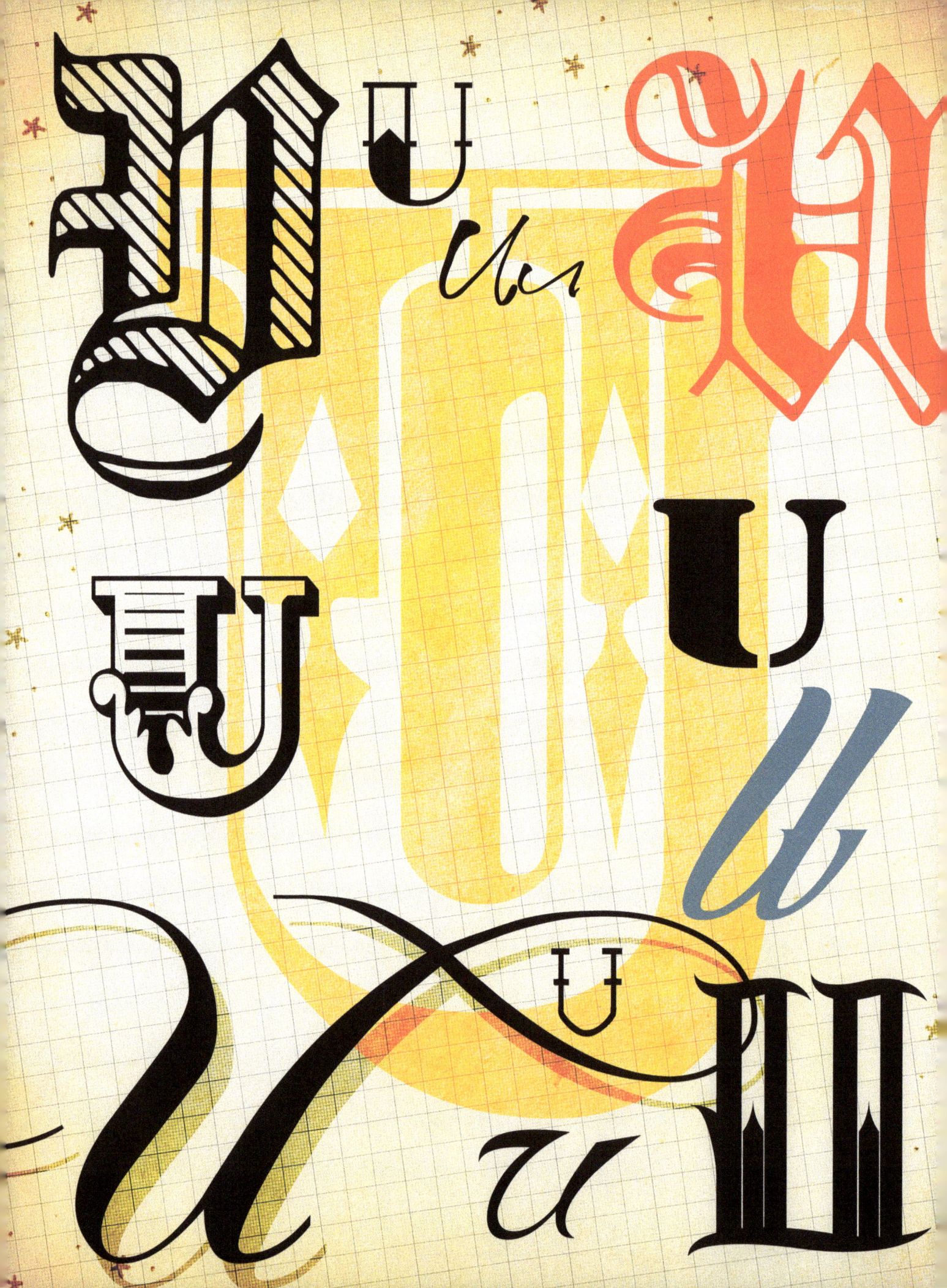

In Loving Memory Of

In Loving Memory Of

In Loving Memory Of

In Loving Memory Of

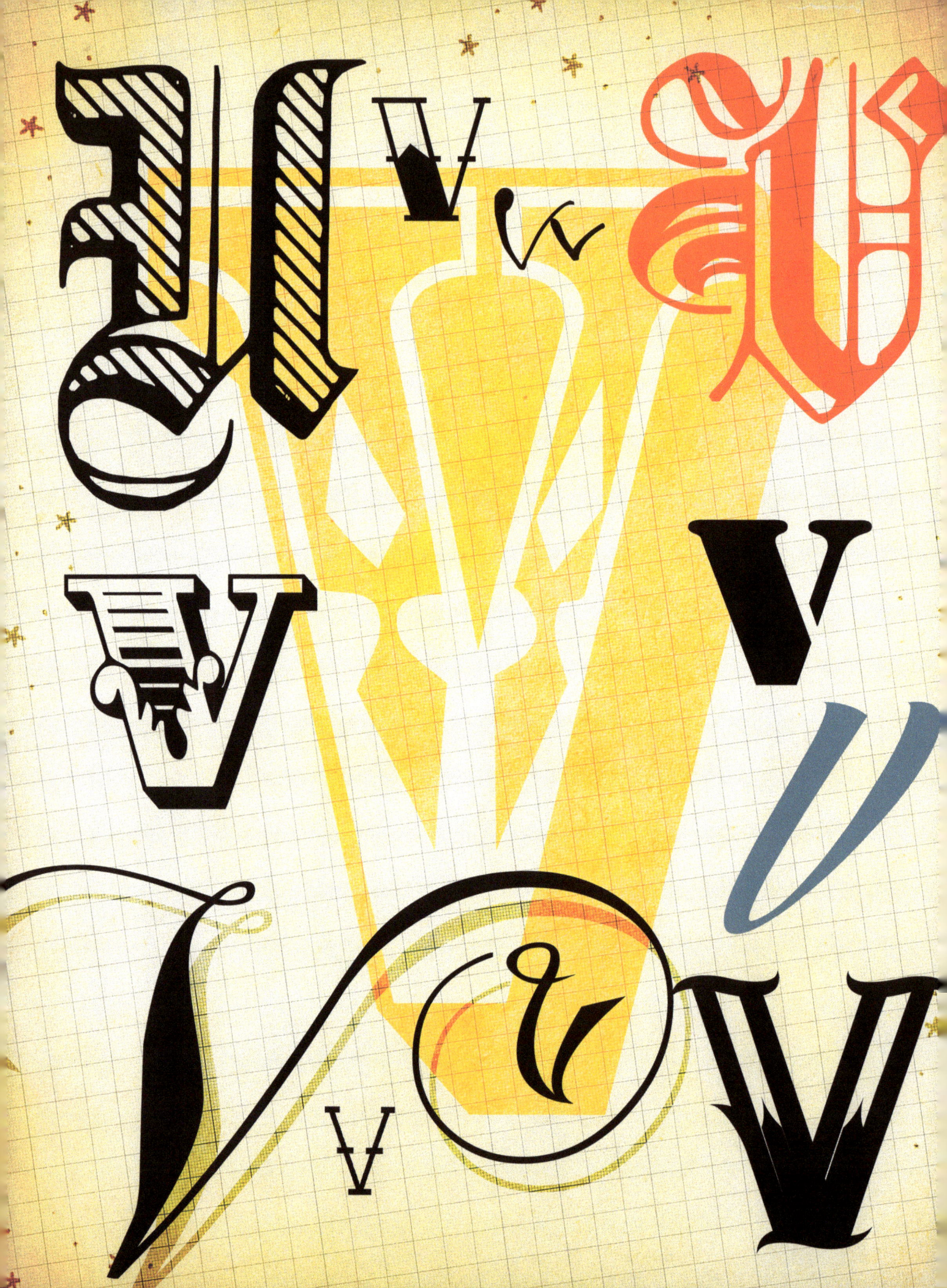

Faith / FAITH / Faith

Faith / Faith / Faith

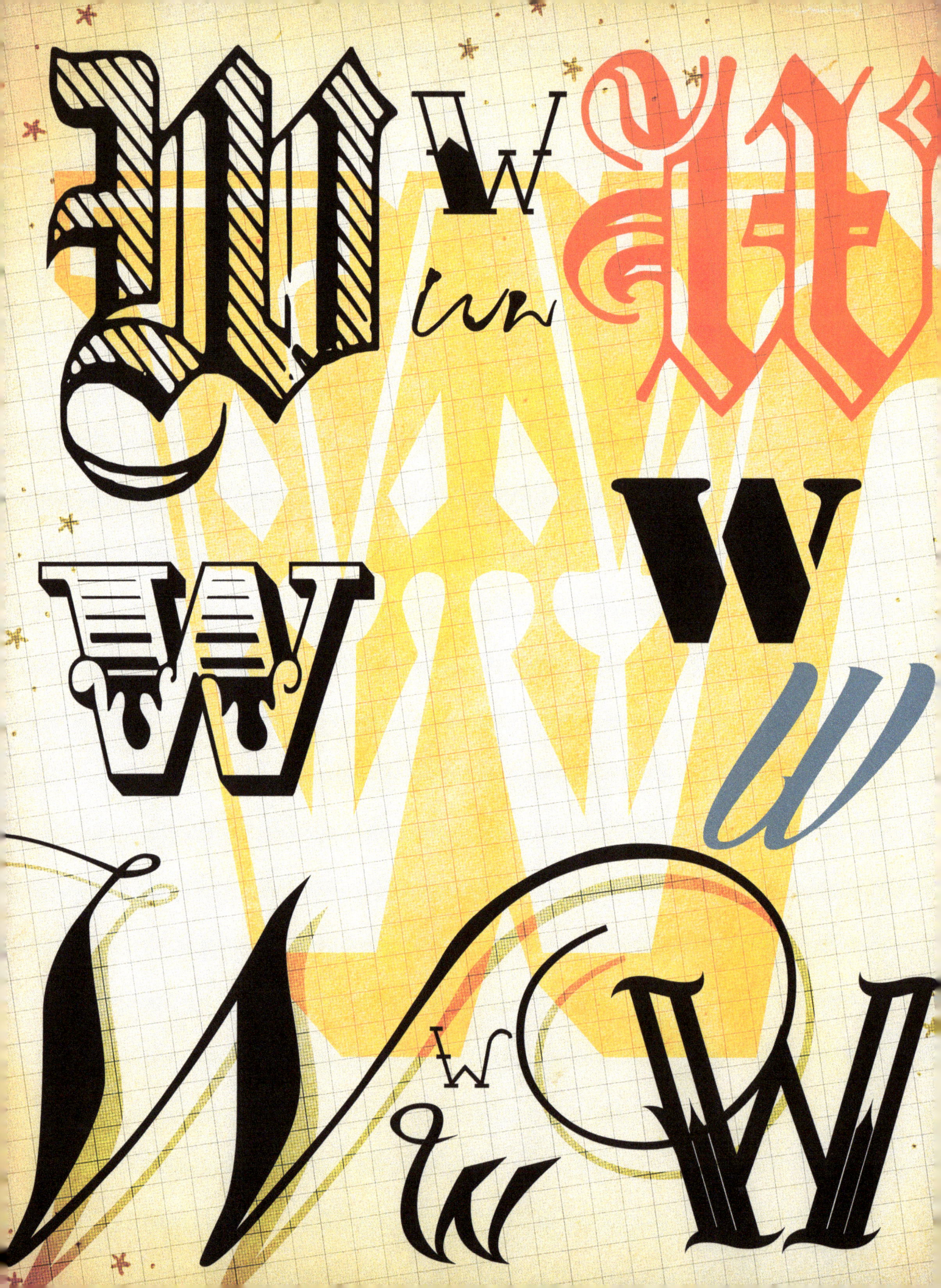

A B C D E F
G H I J K L
M N O P Q R S
T U V W X Y Z

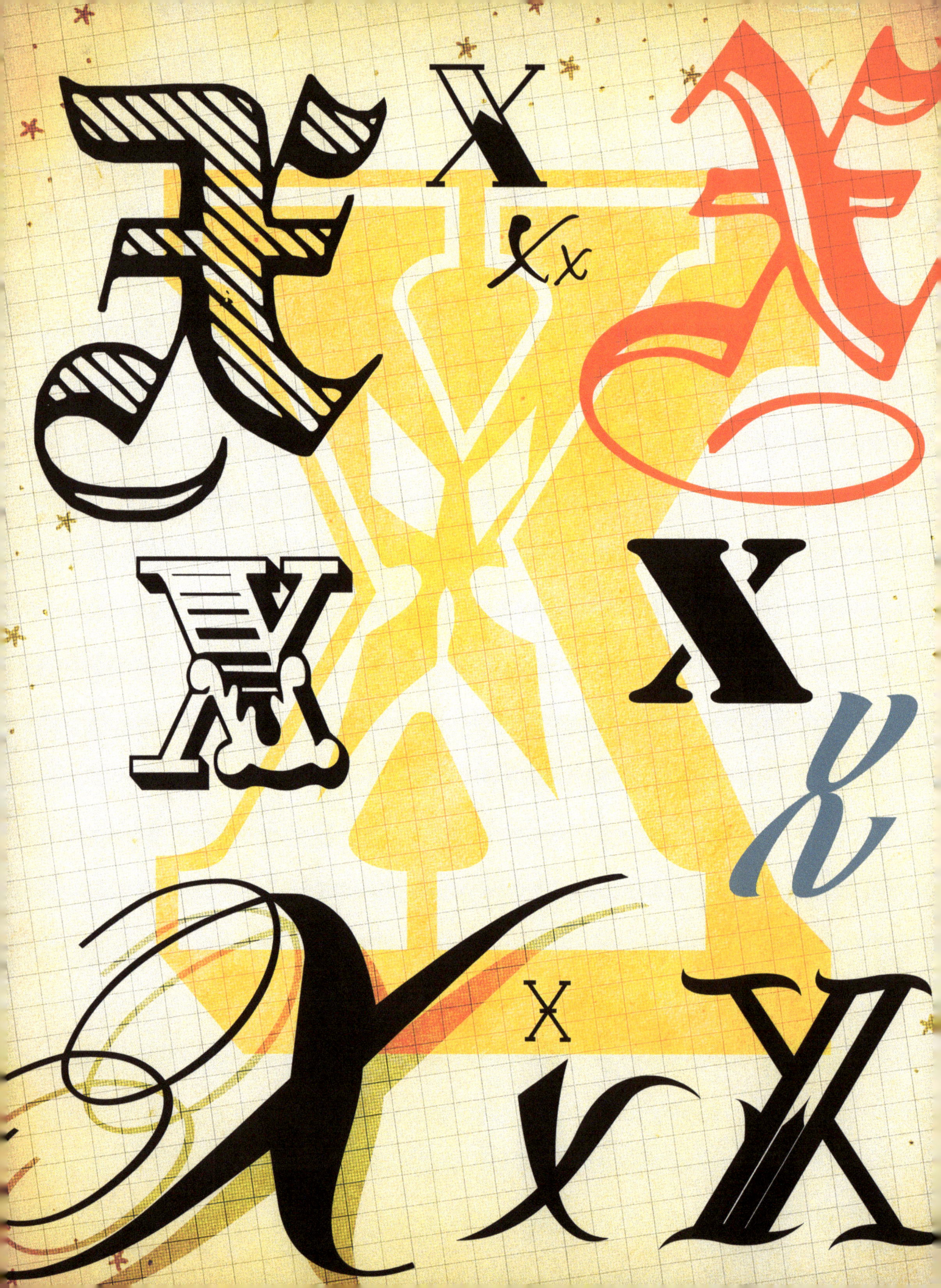

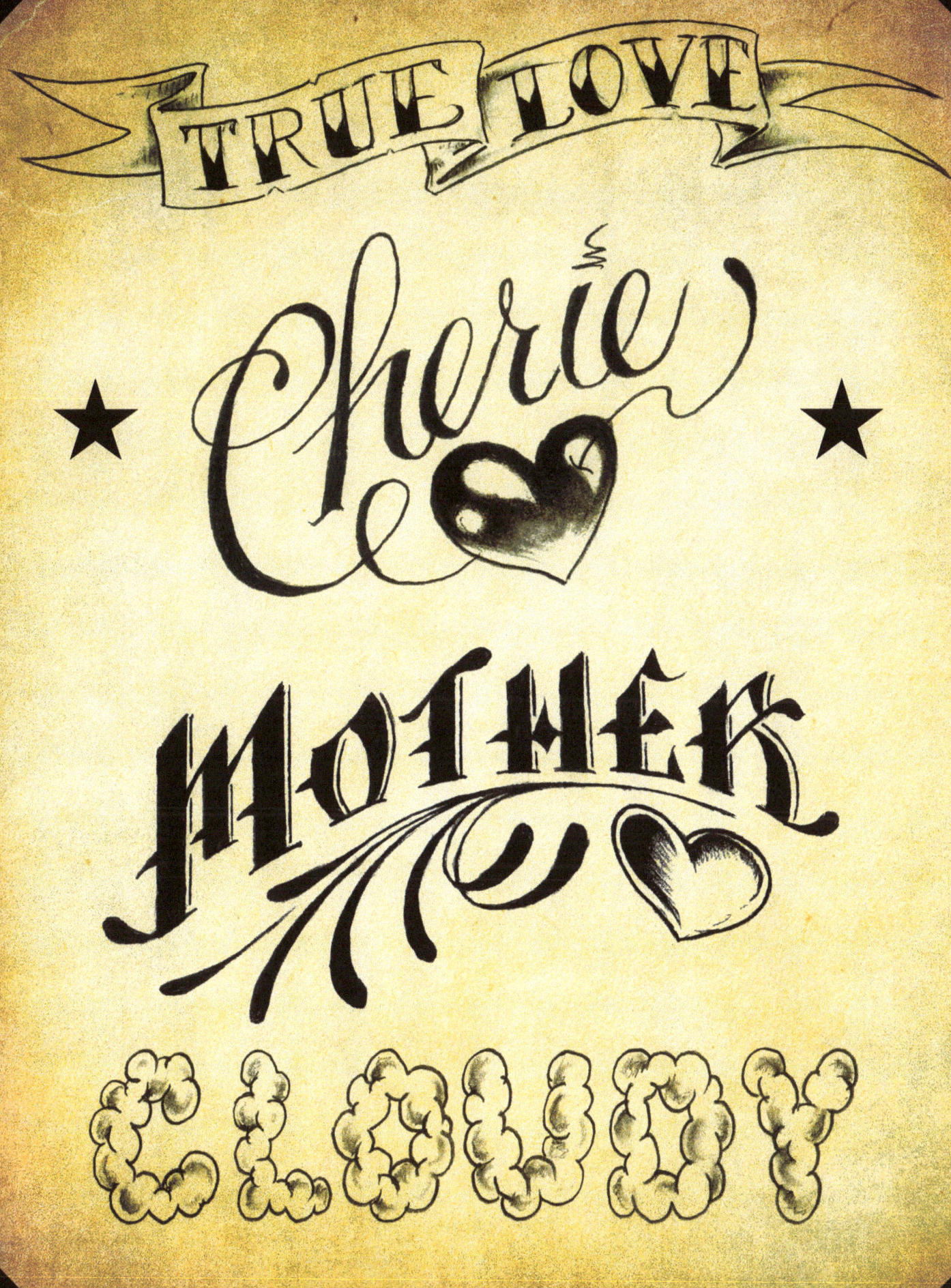

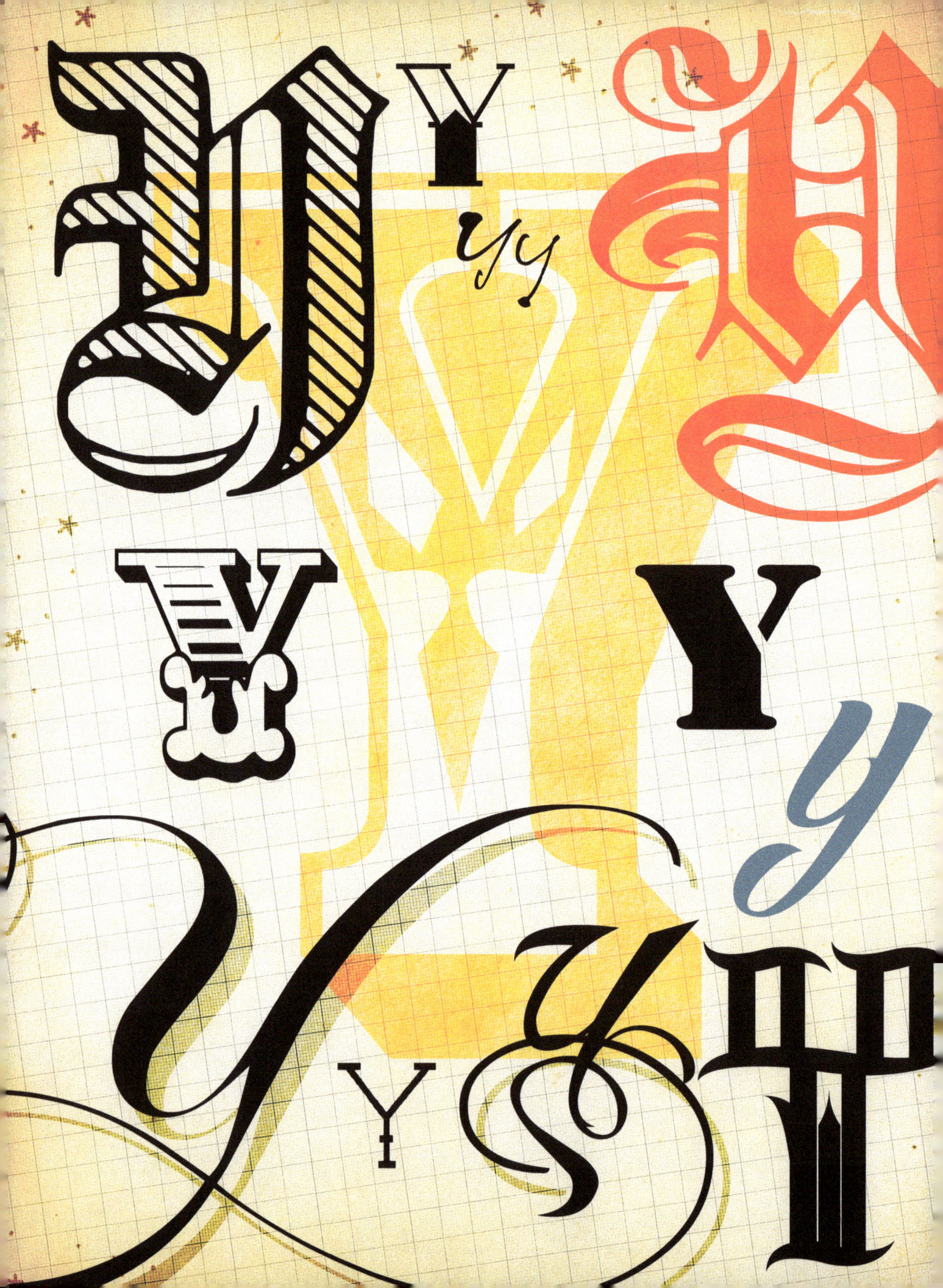

JUSTINE

PIS

ABCDEFG
HIJKLM
NOPQRST
UVWXYZ

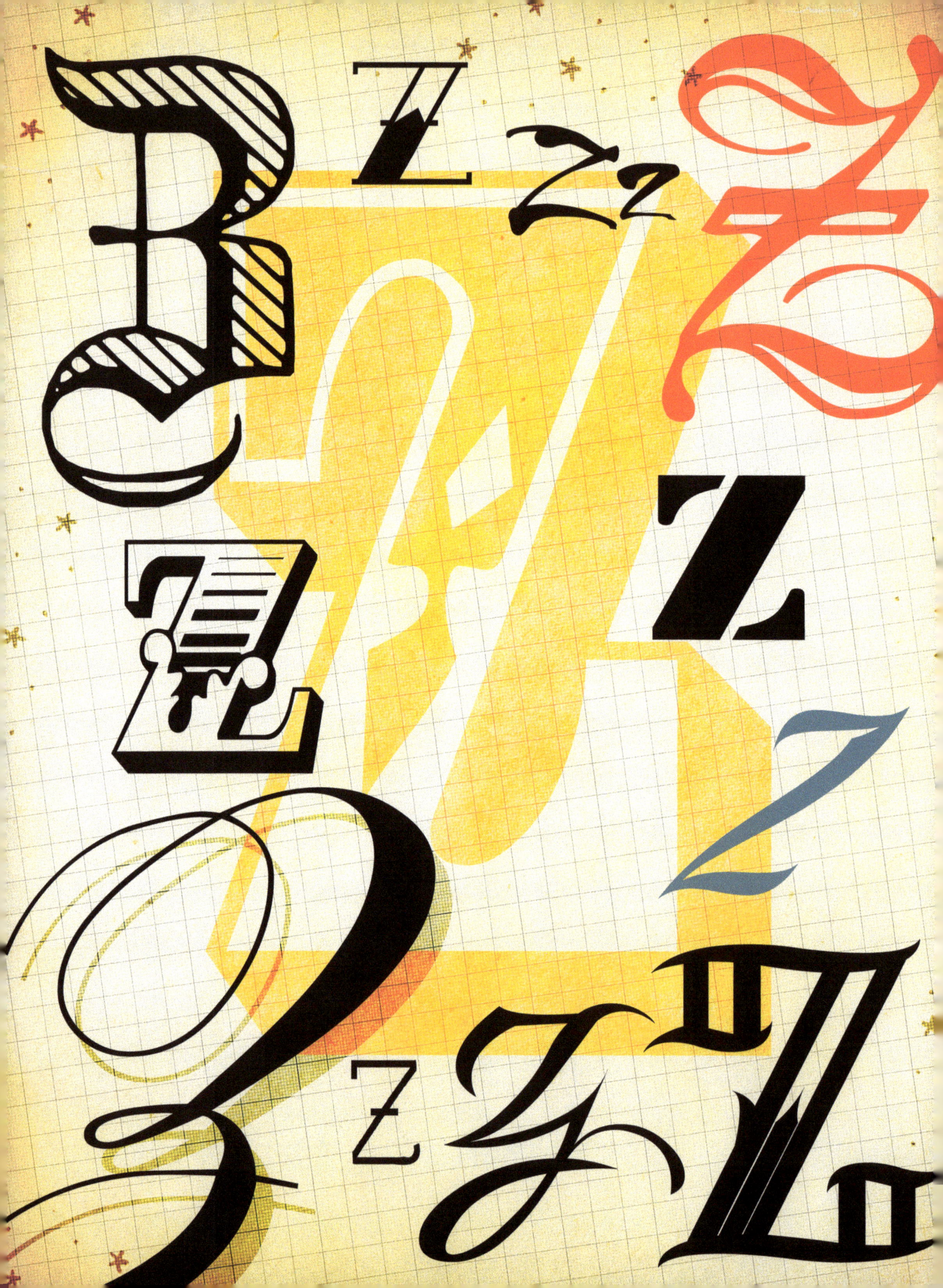

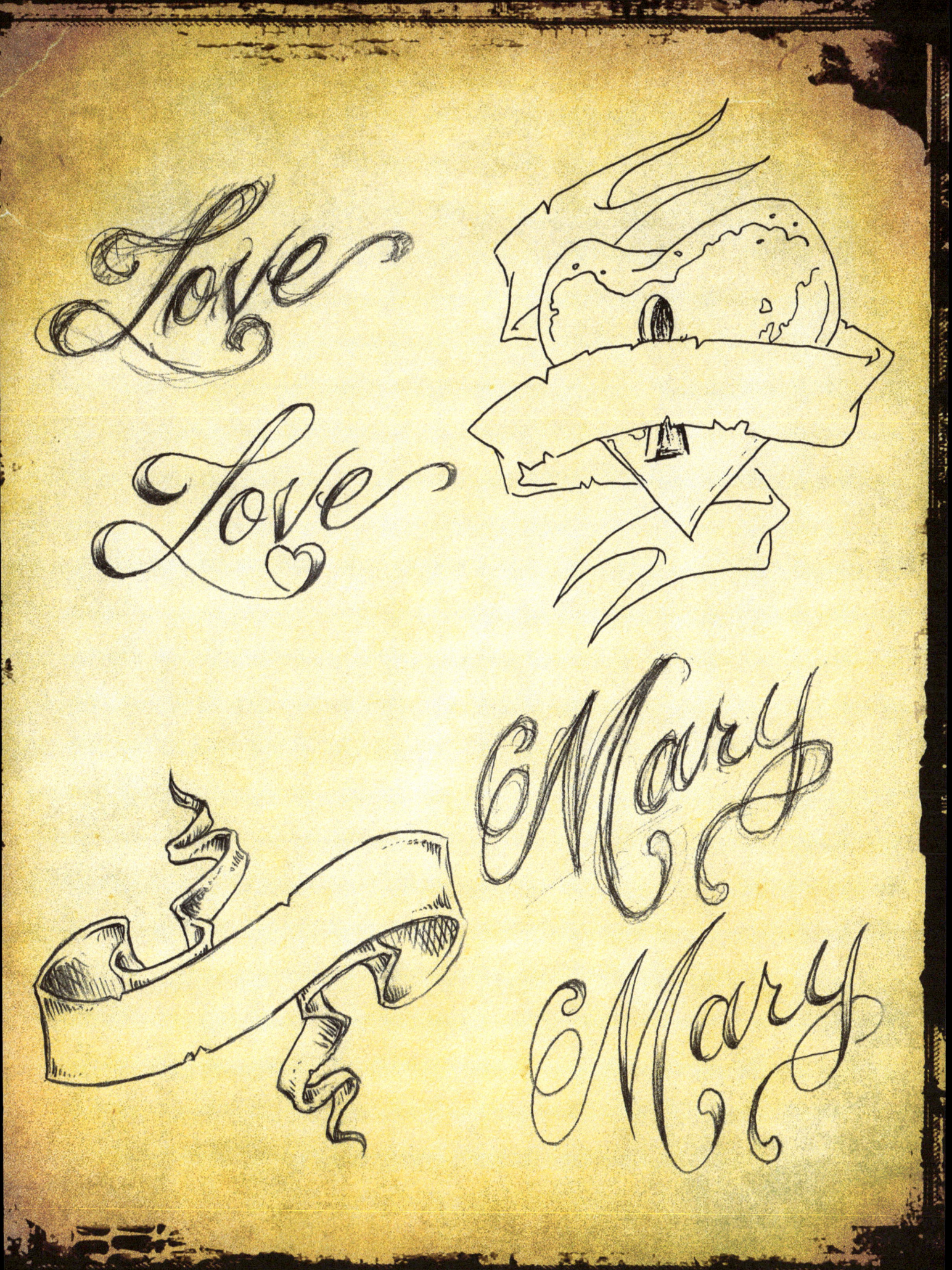

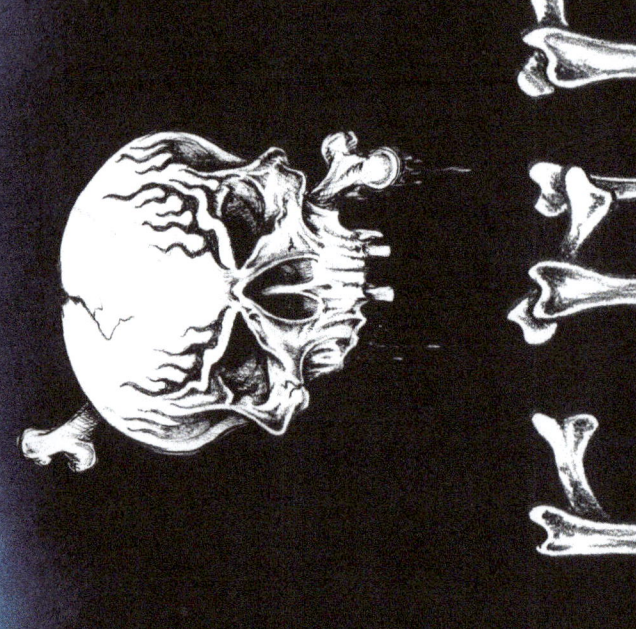

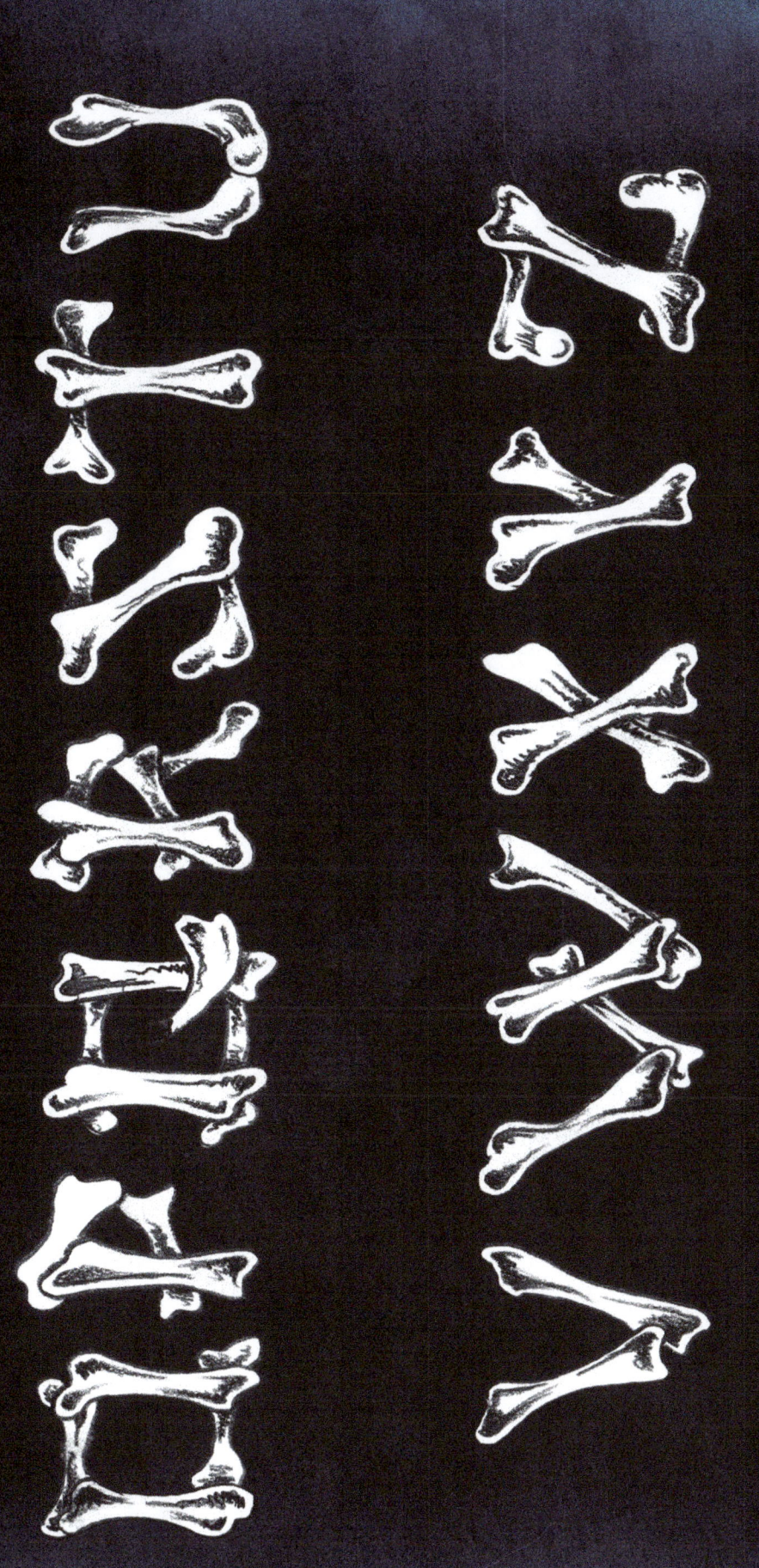

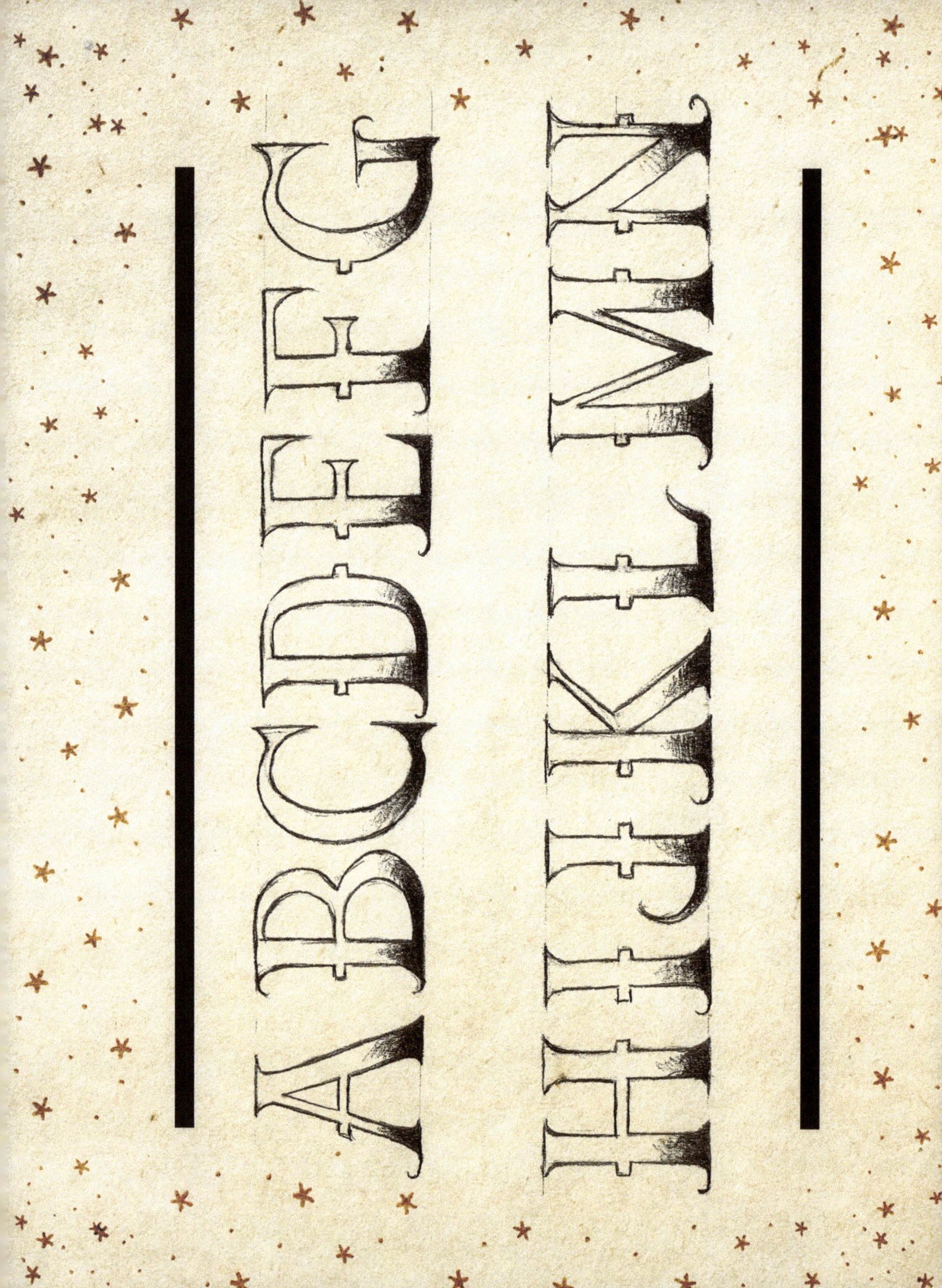

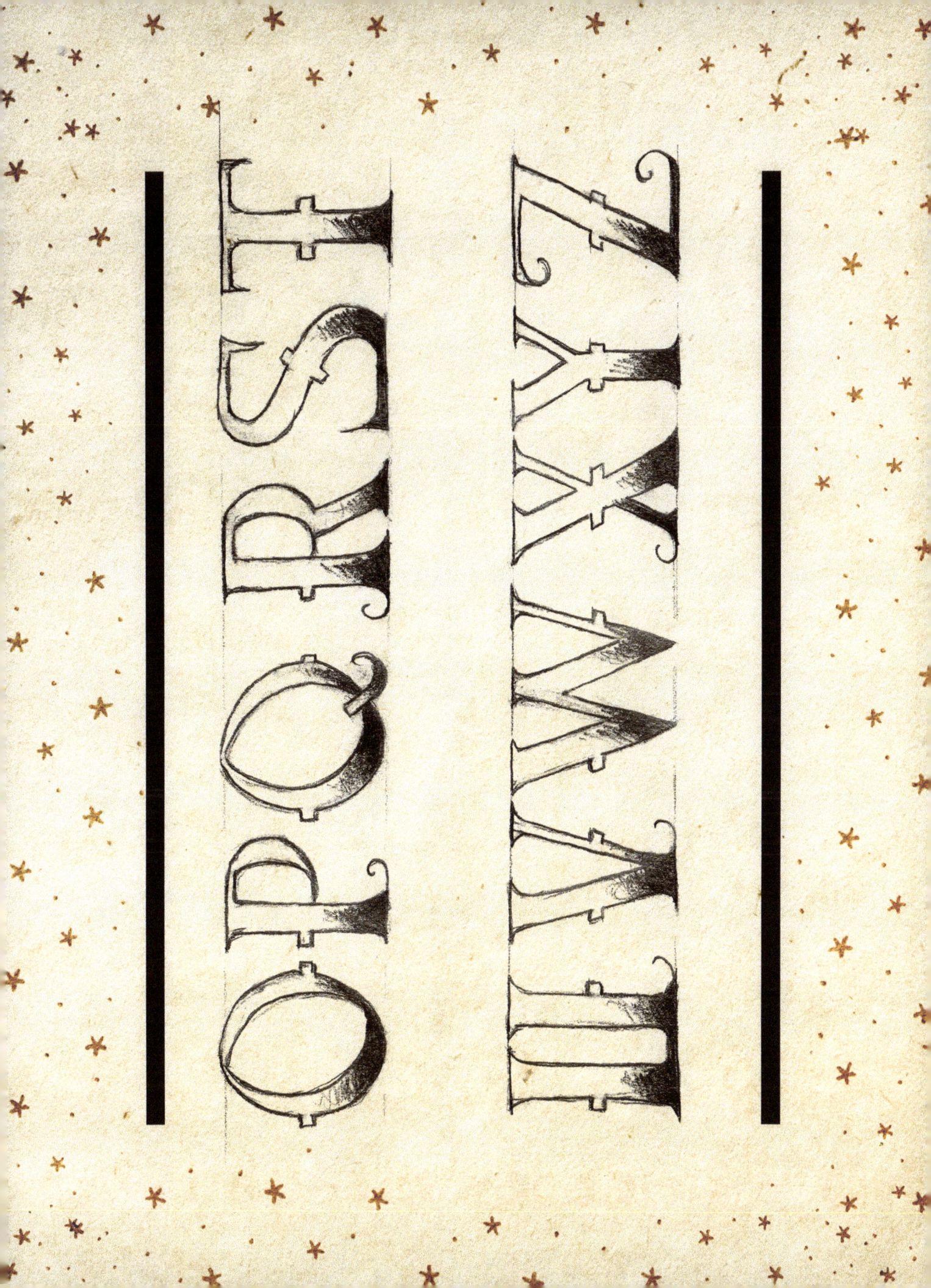

ONE
PLUS
ONE
EQUALS
ABC

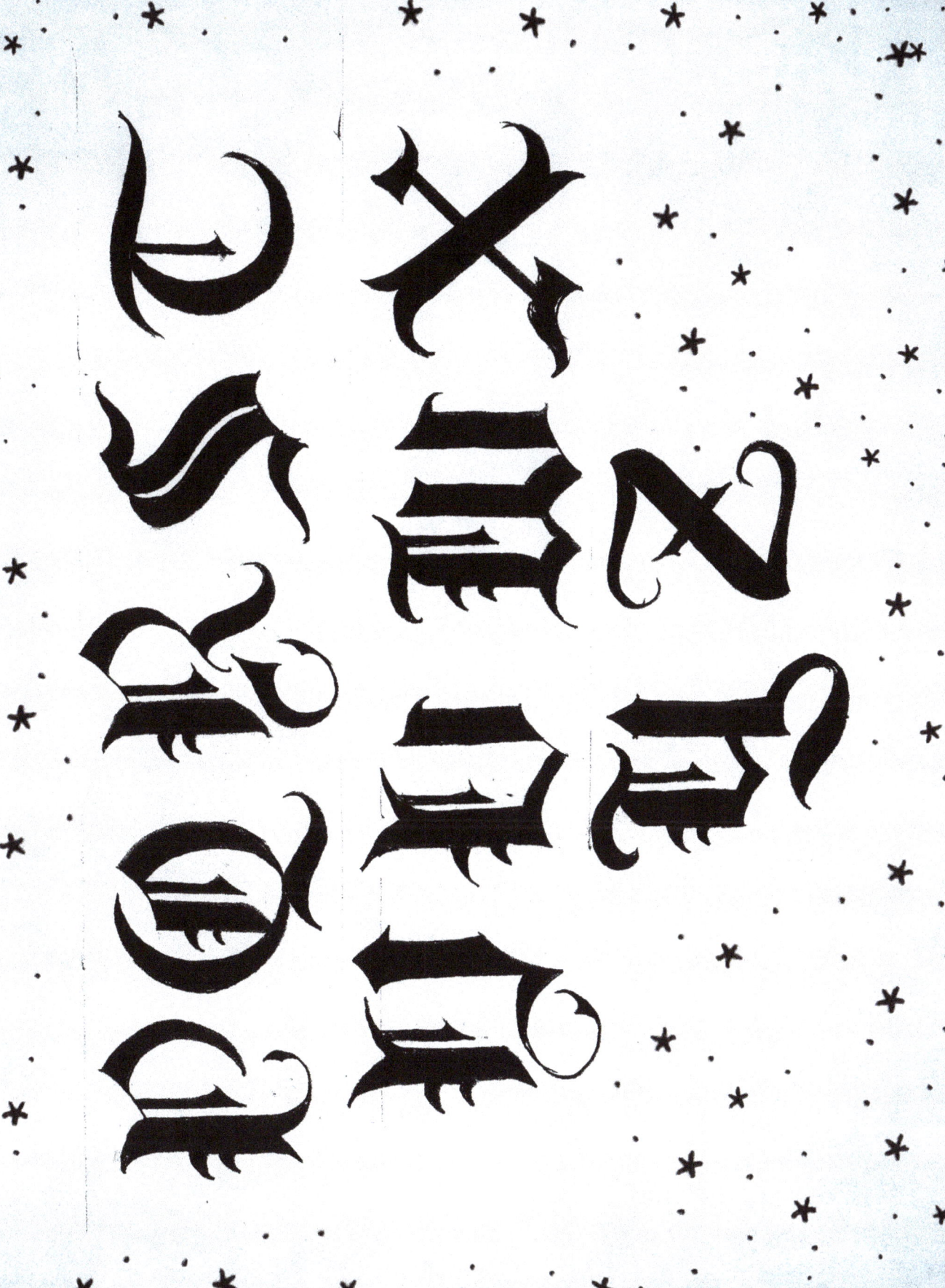

Smile Now Cry Later

Smile Now Cry Later

Smile Now Cry Later

Smile Now Cry Later

★ HOME ★

ABCDEFGHIJKL
MNOPQRSTU
VWXYZ

A B C D E F G

H I J K L M N

OPQRST UVWXYZ

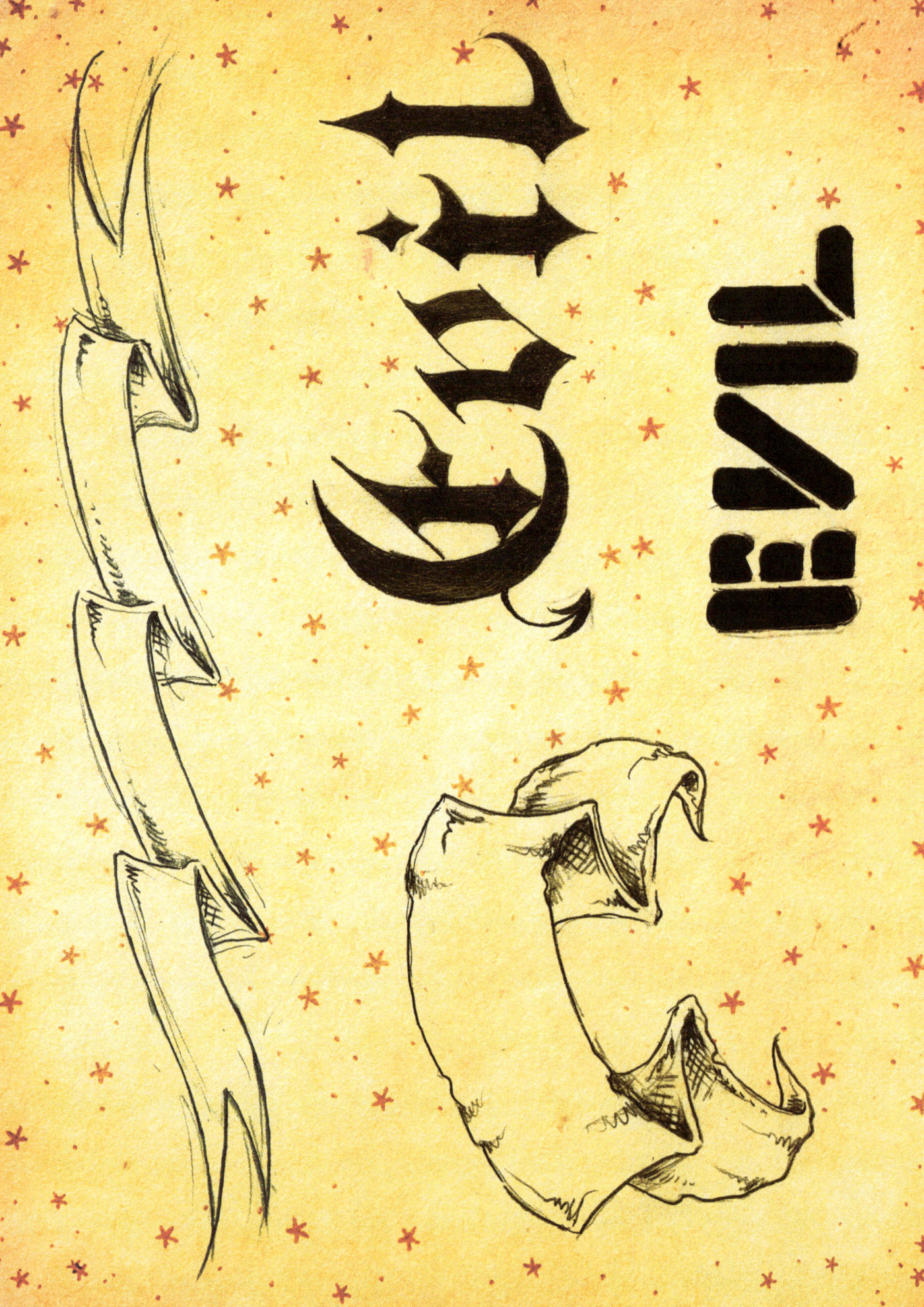

God God God

God God God

AaBbCcDd
EeFfGgHh
IiJjKkLlMmNn
OoPpQqRrSsTt
UuVvWwXxYyZz

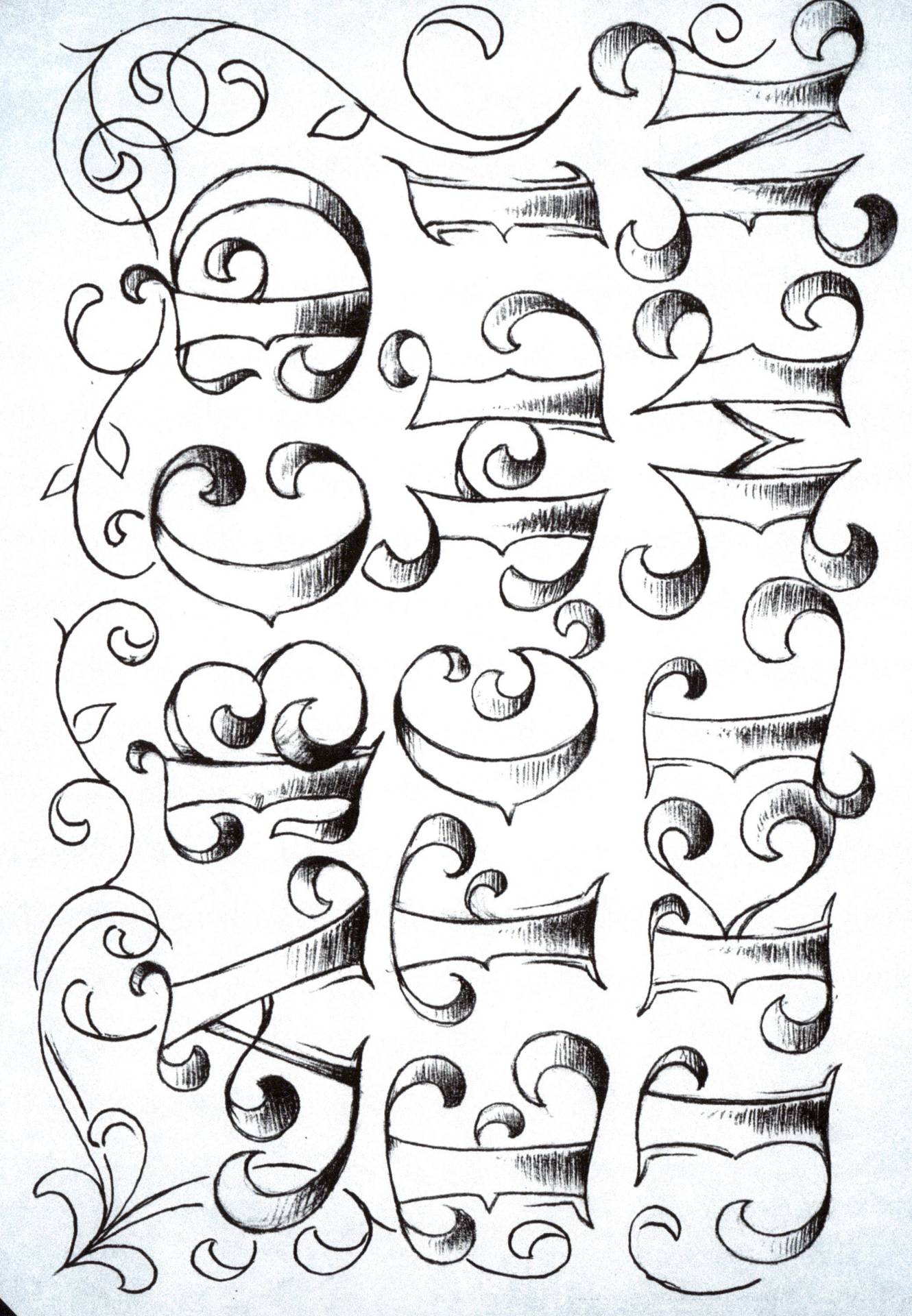

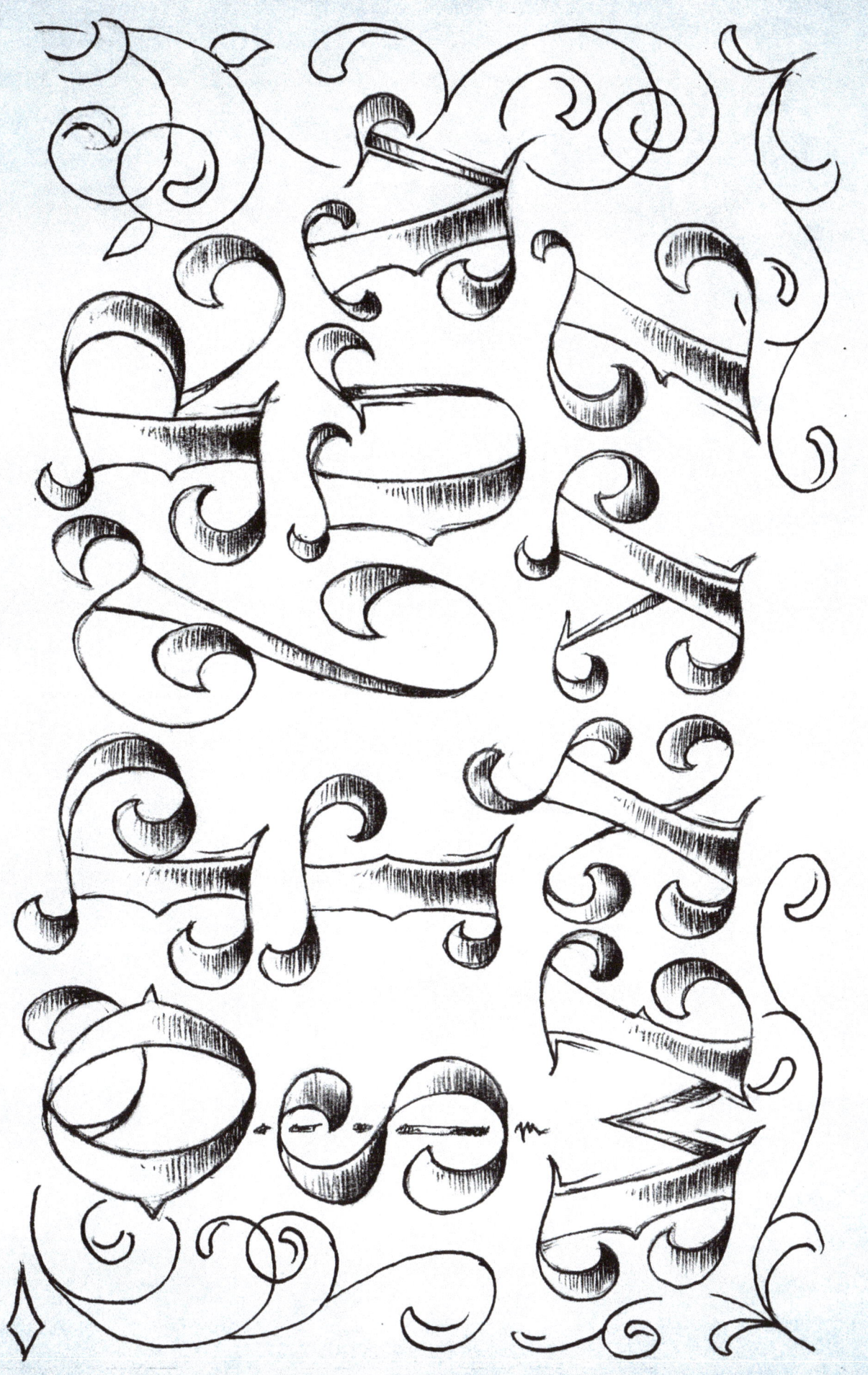

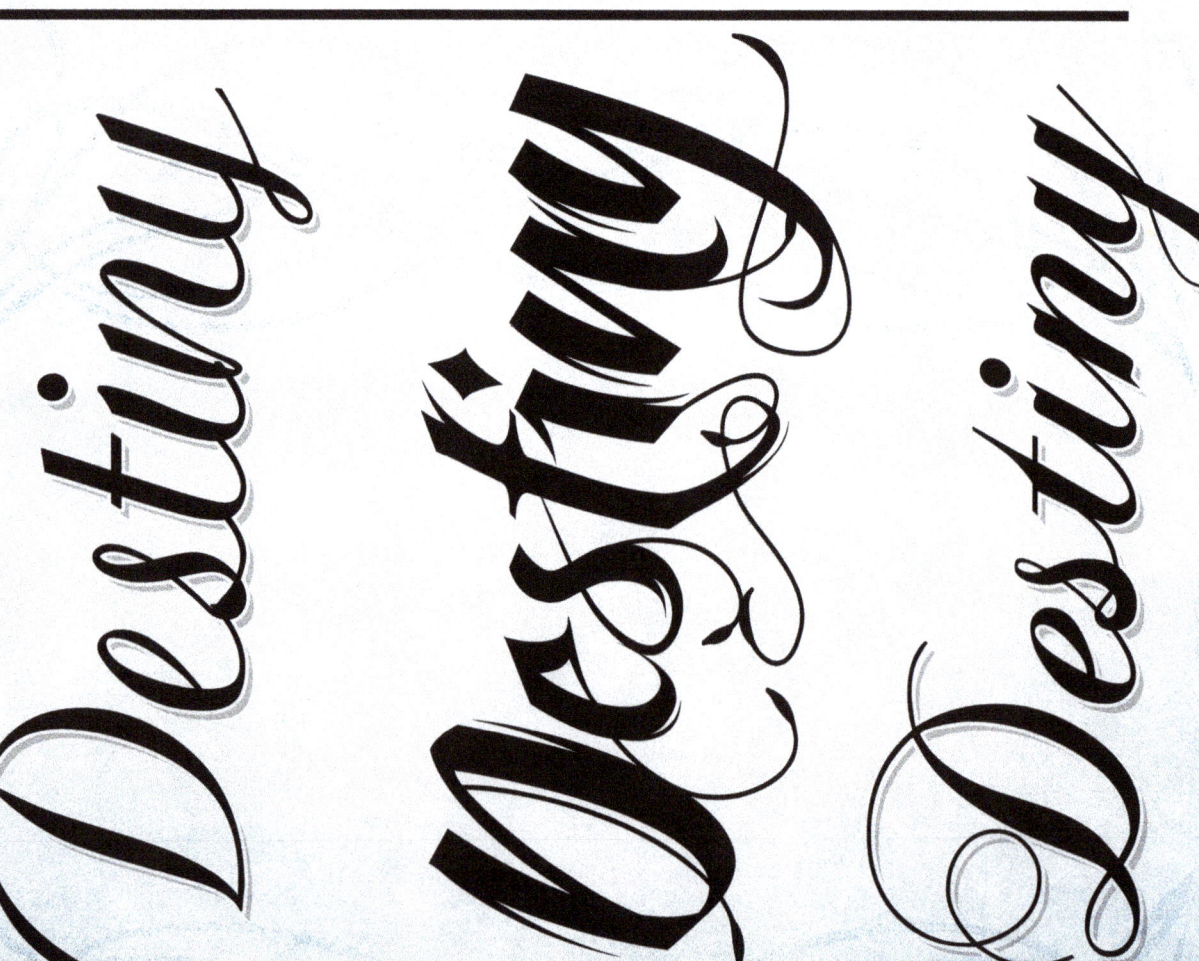

ABCDE
FGHIJ
KLMNO
PQRST
UVWX
YZ

Smile Smile Smile

Smile Smile Smile

You Only Live Once

You Only Live Once

You Only Live Once

You Only Live Once

ABCDEFG
HIJKLMN
OPQRST
UVWXYZ

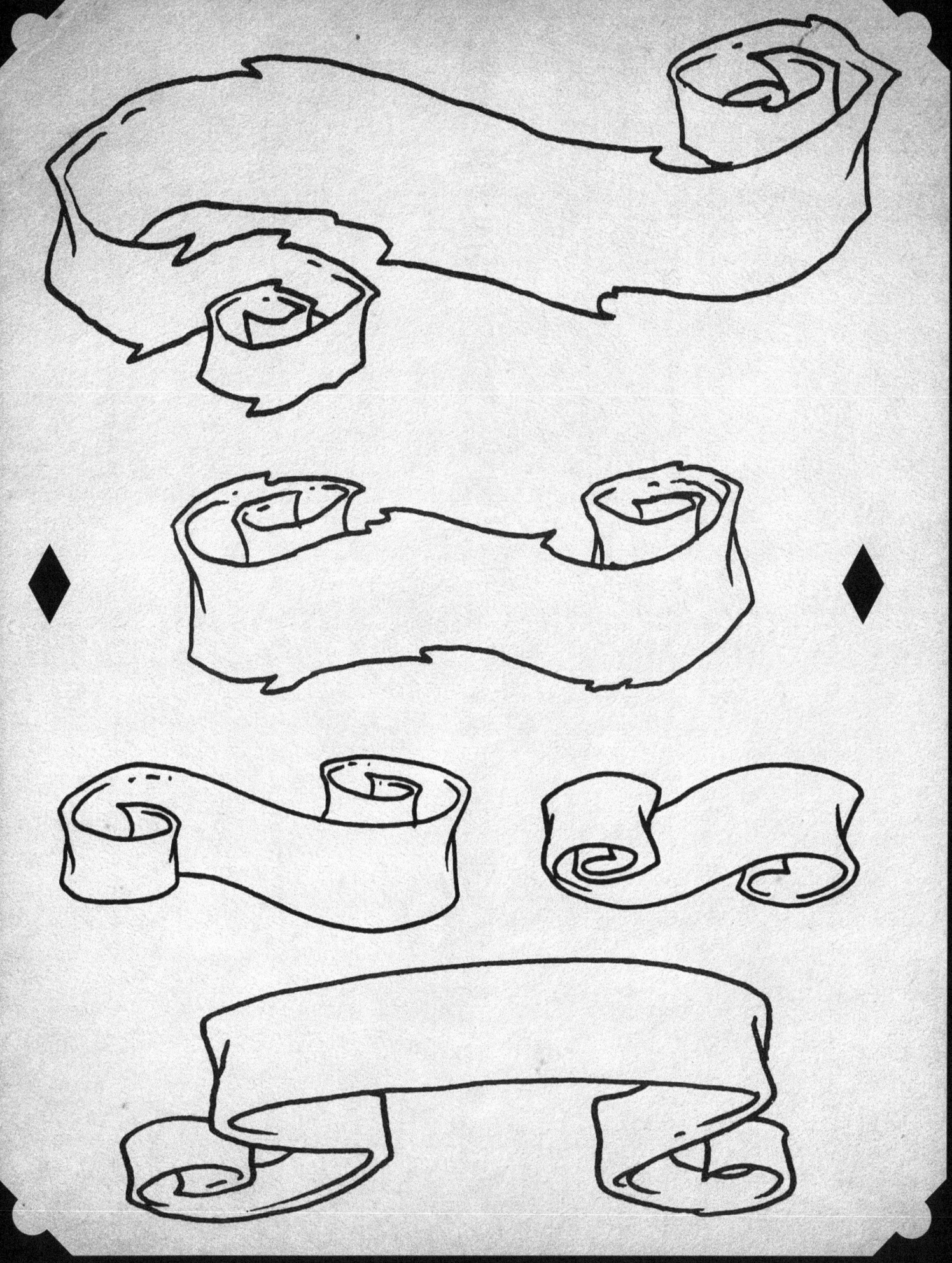

abcdefghijkl
mnopqrstuvw
xyz

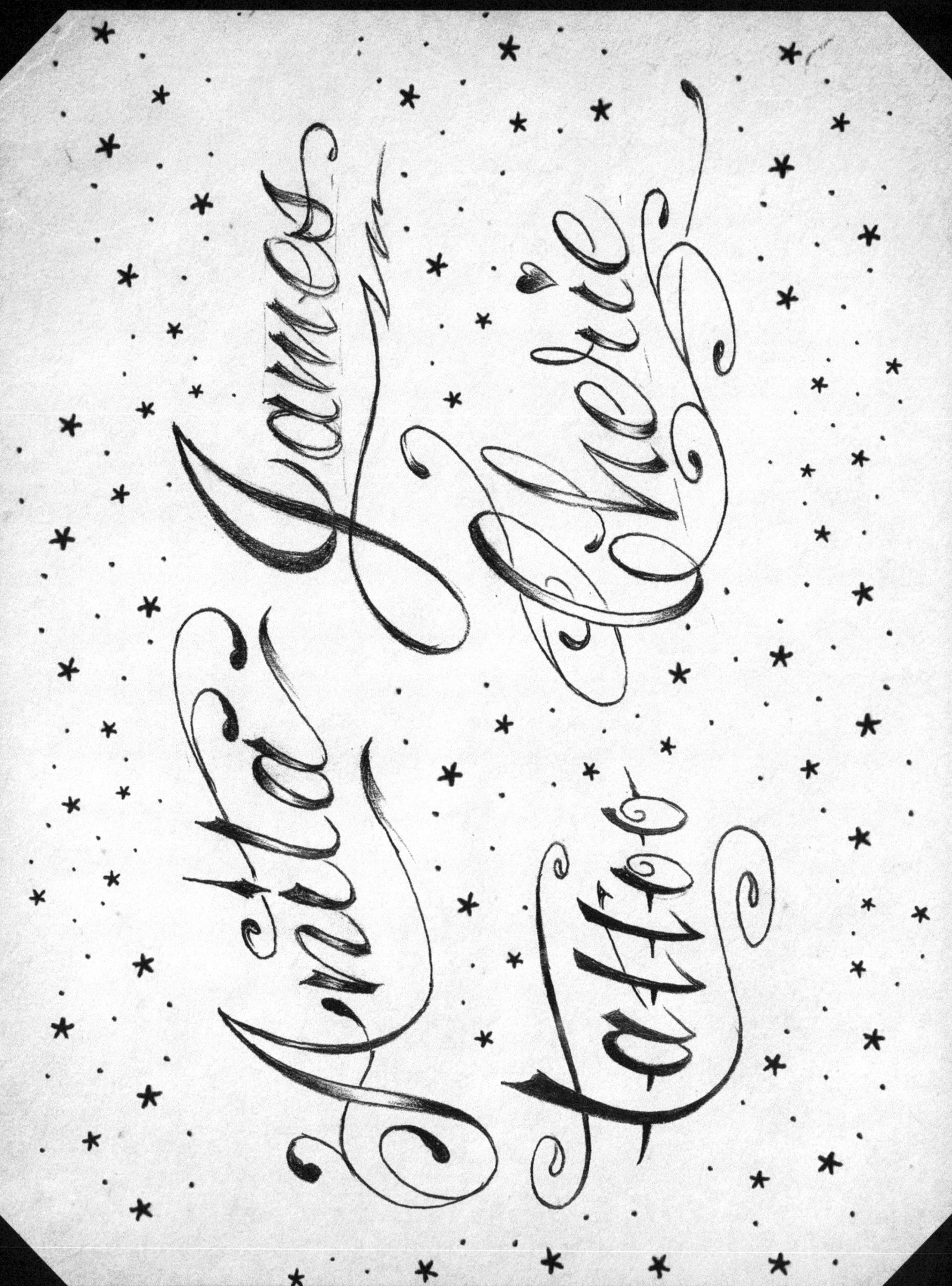

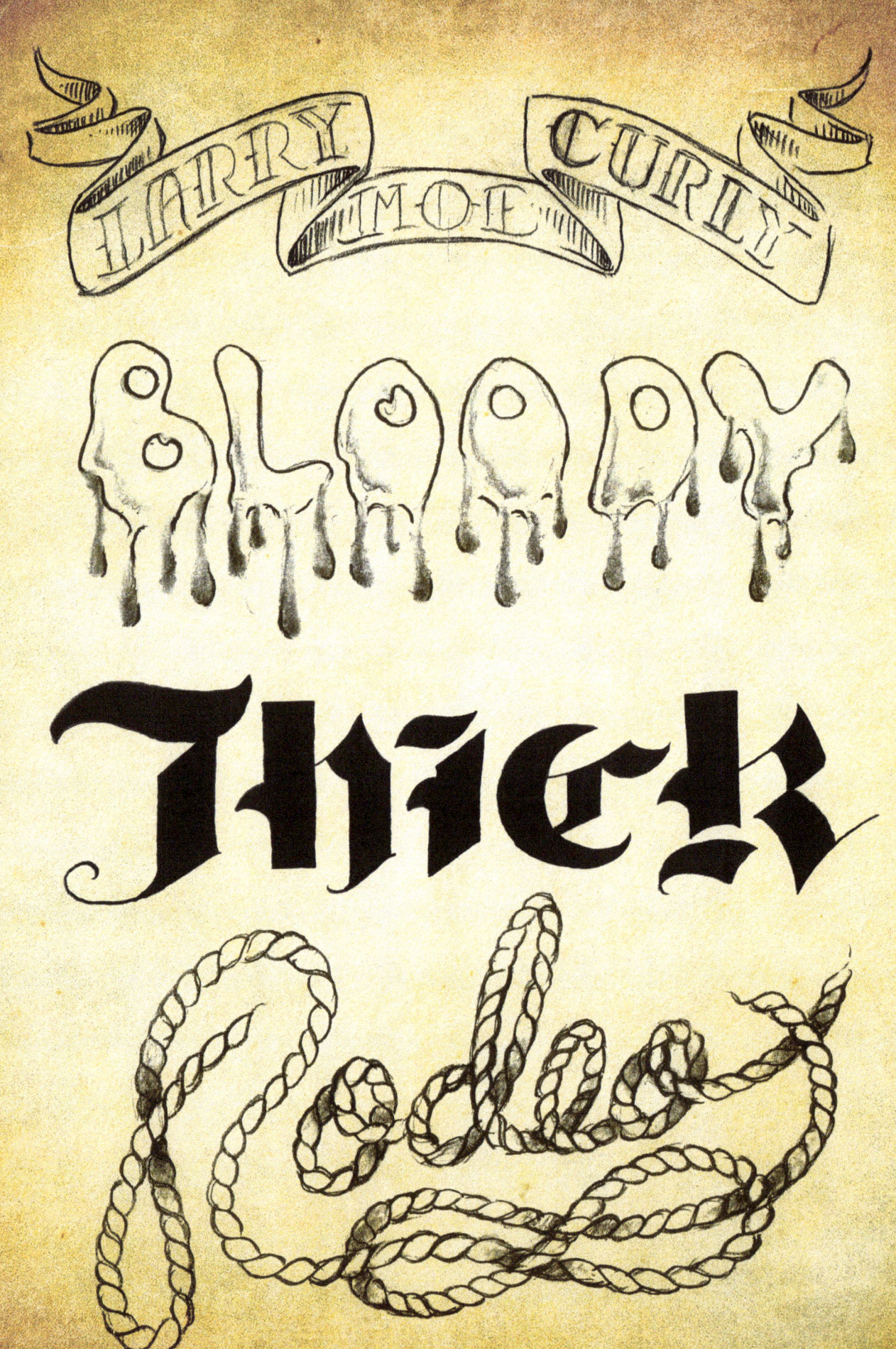

HAWAII

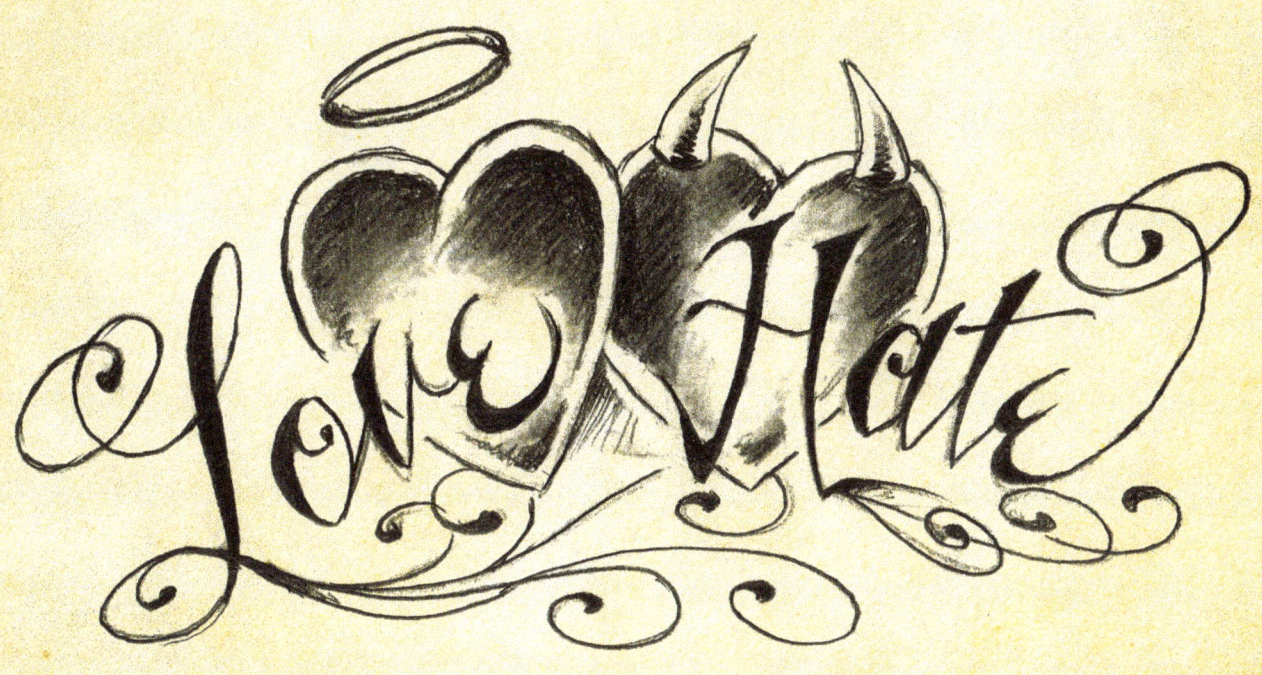

GOTHIC

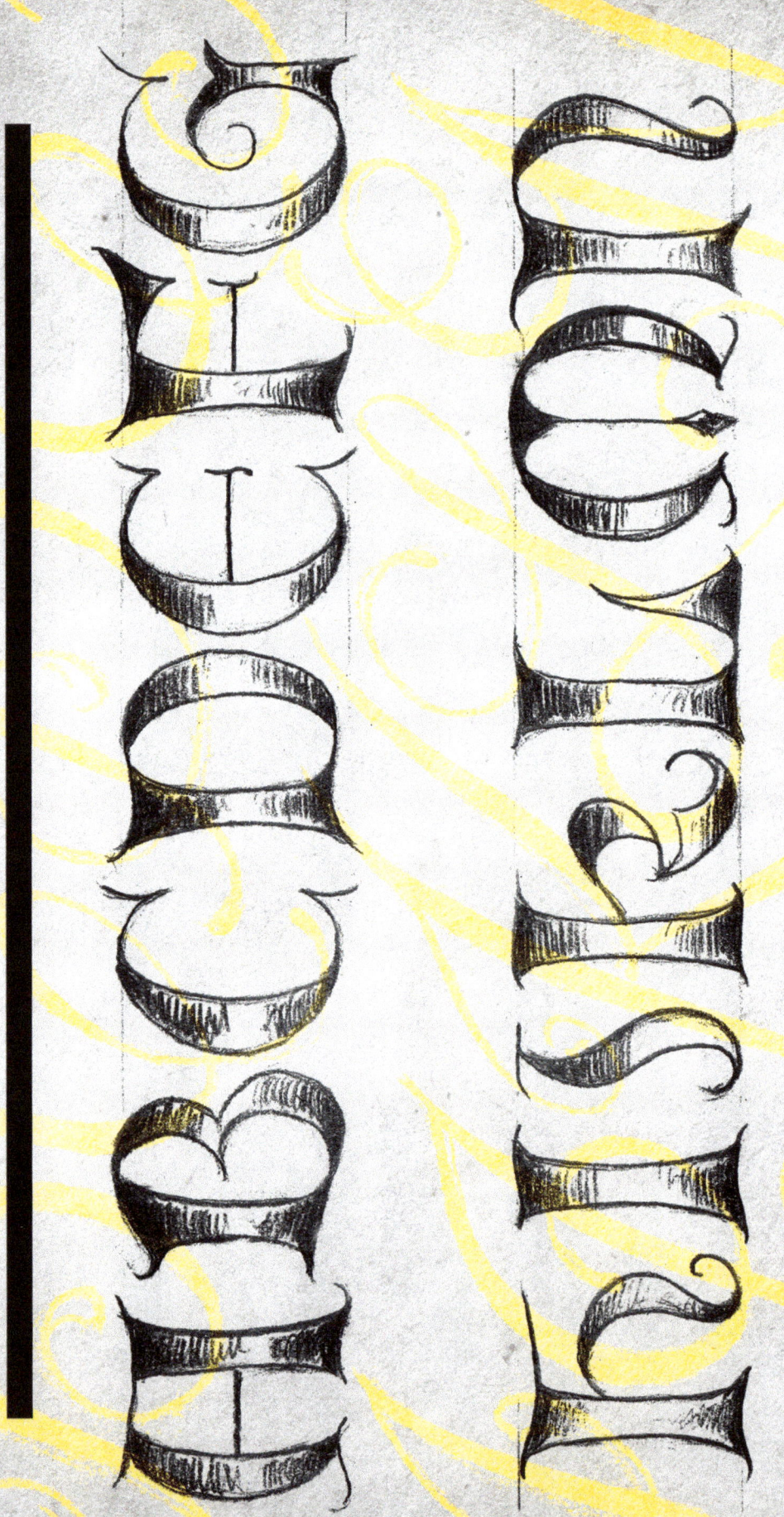

OPEN MIND

Hope HOPE Hope

Hope Hope Hope

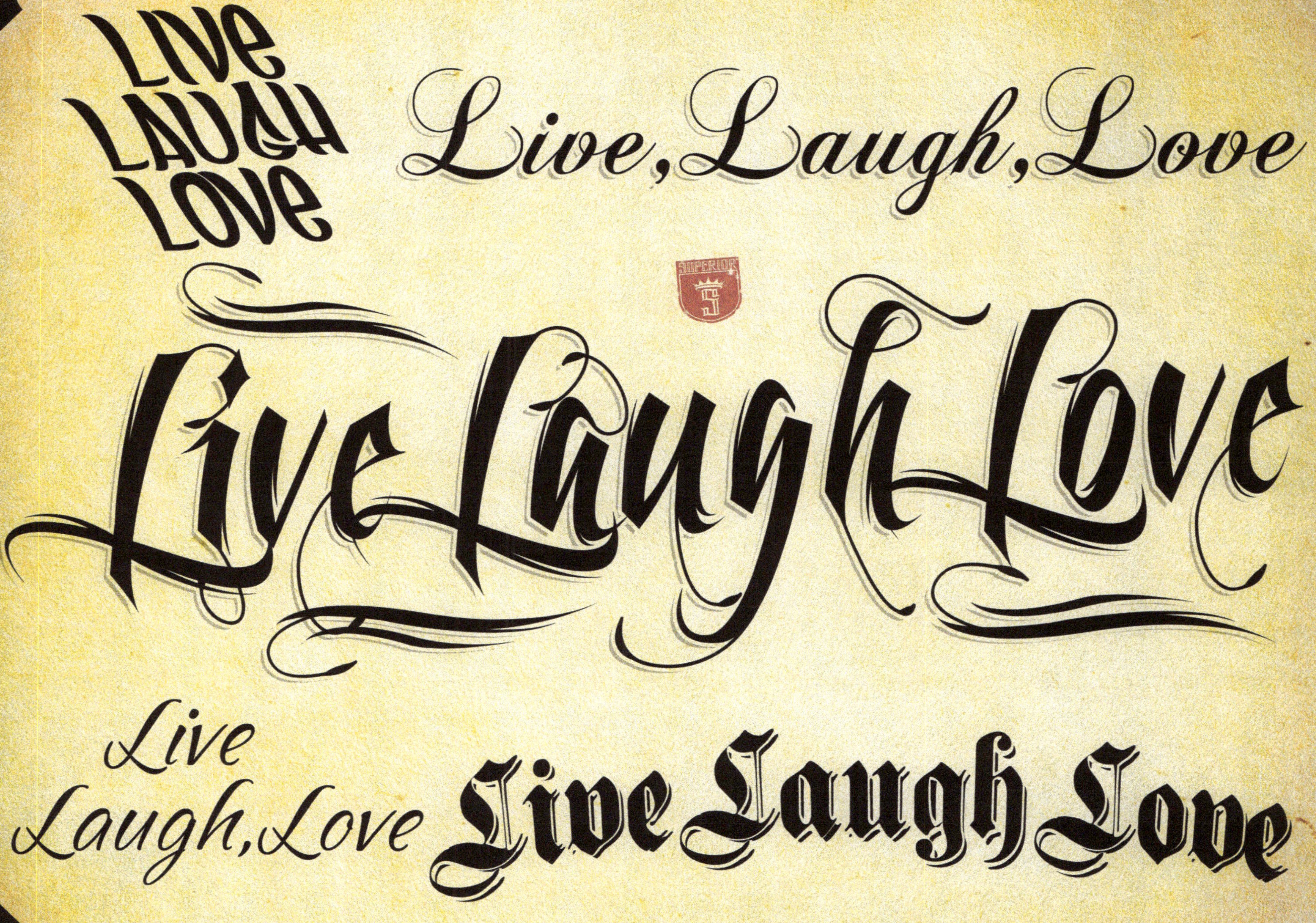

Live, Laugh, Love

Live Laugh Love

Live Laugh Love

Live Love Laugh

LIVE LAUGH LOVE

Live Laugh, Love

A B C D E F G H I J K L M N O P Q R S T U V W X Y Z

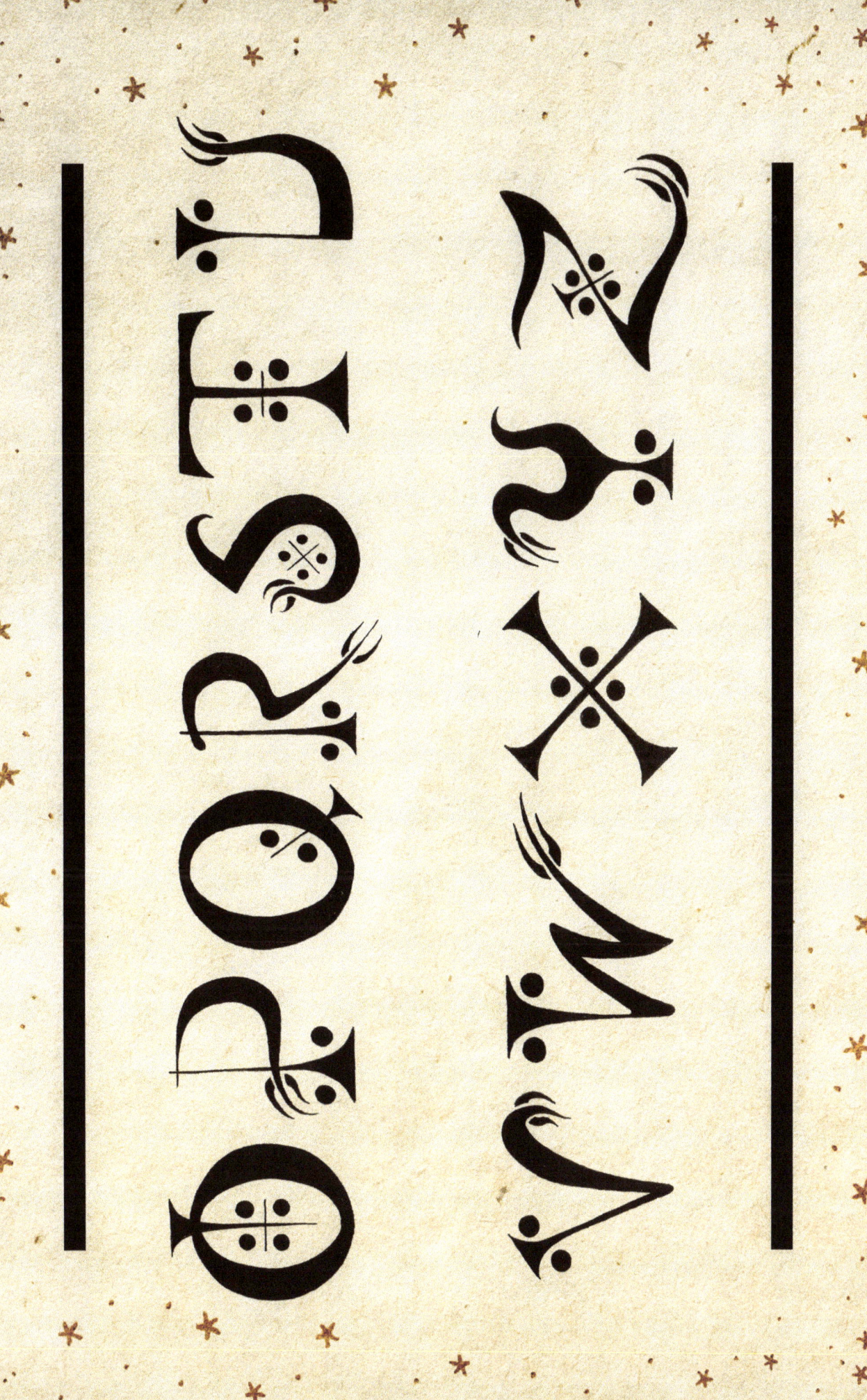

My Brother's Keeper

My Brother's Keeper

My Brother's Keeper

My Brother's Keeper

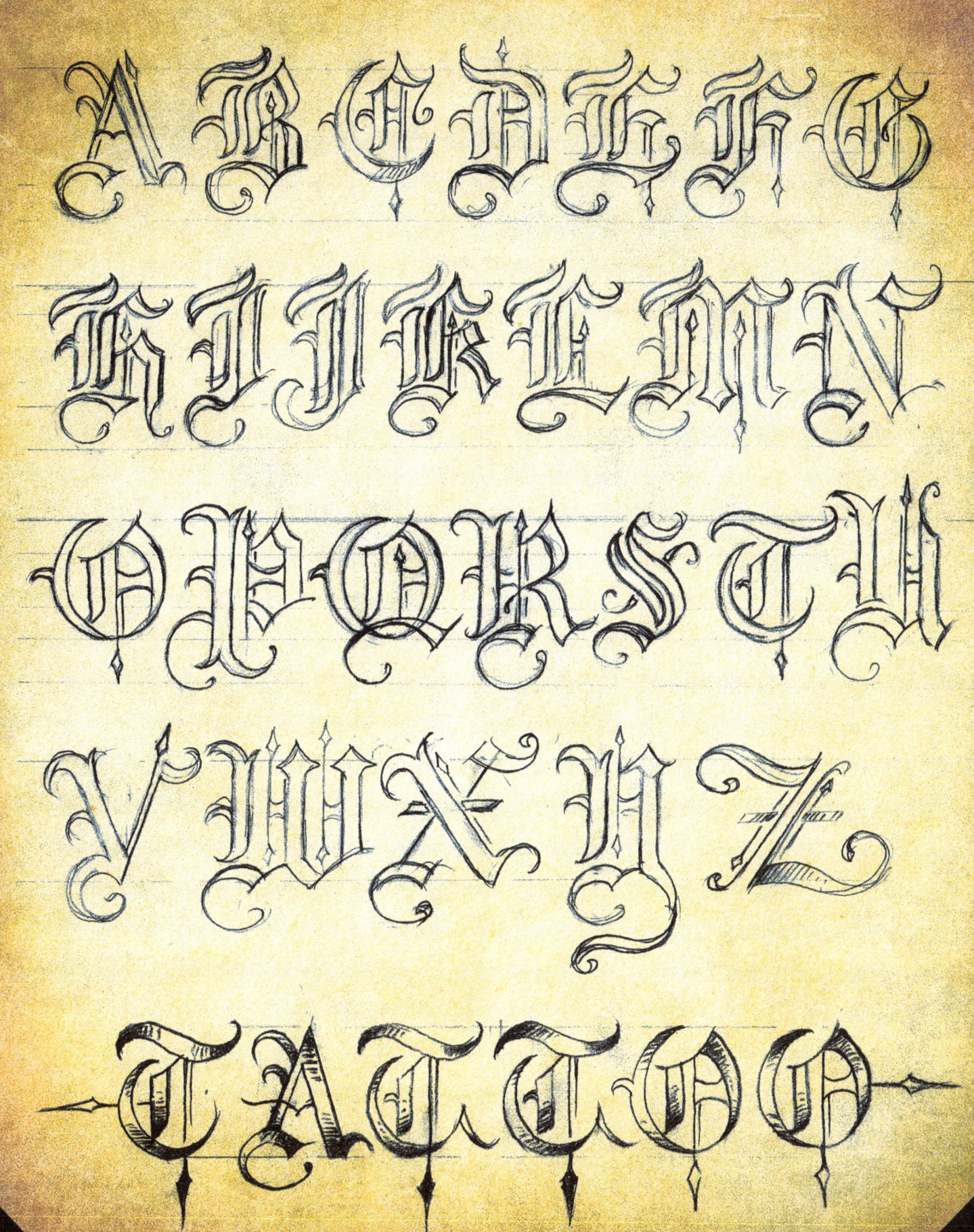

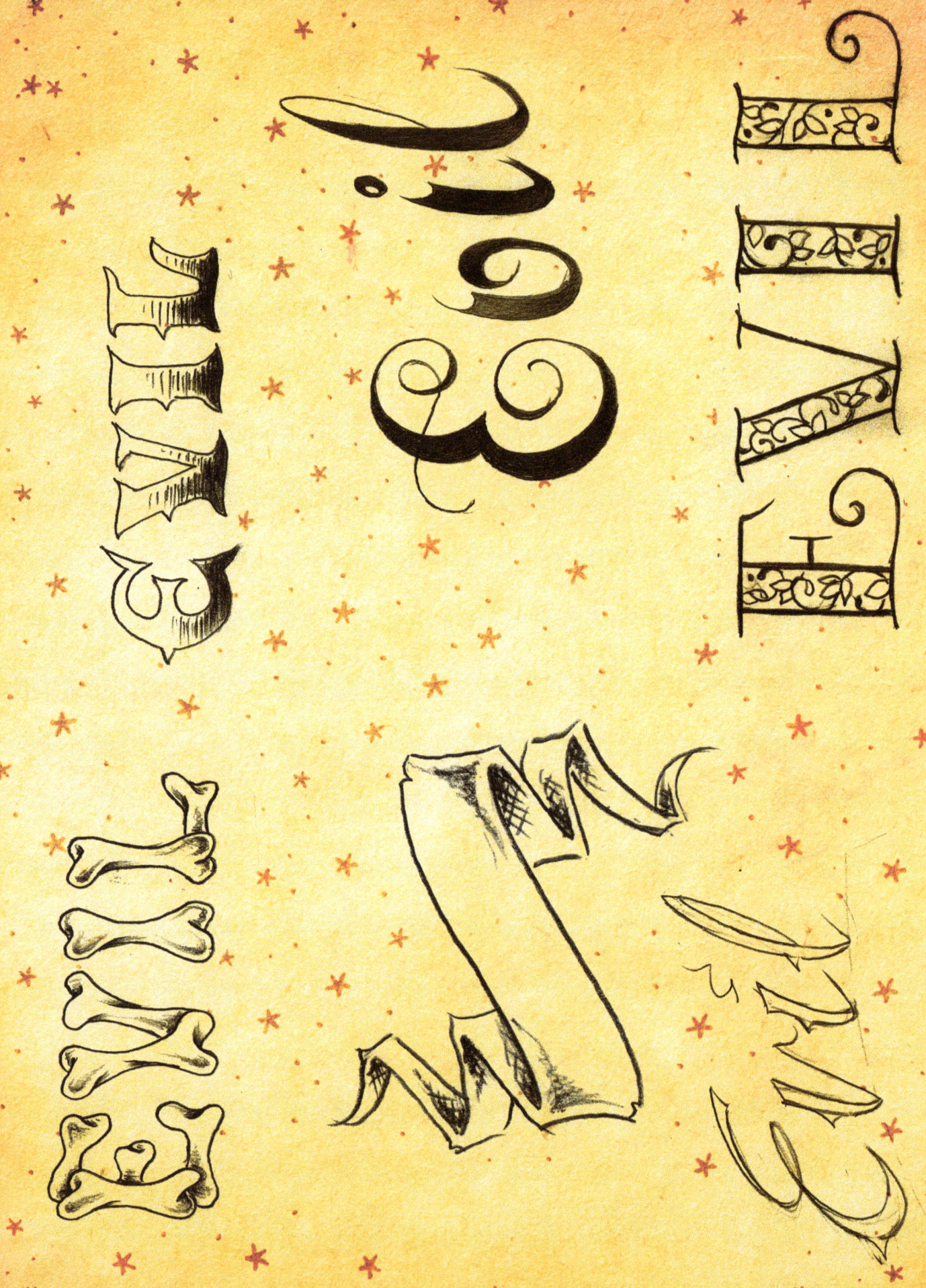

Fate / FATE / Fate

Fate / Fate / Fate

Conquer Conquer Conquer

Conquer Conquer Conquer

- Always Forgive Never Forget
- Always Forgive Never Forget
- Always Forgive Never Forget
- Always Forgive Never Forget

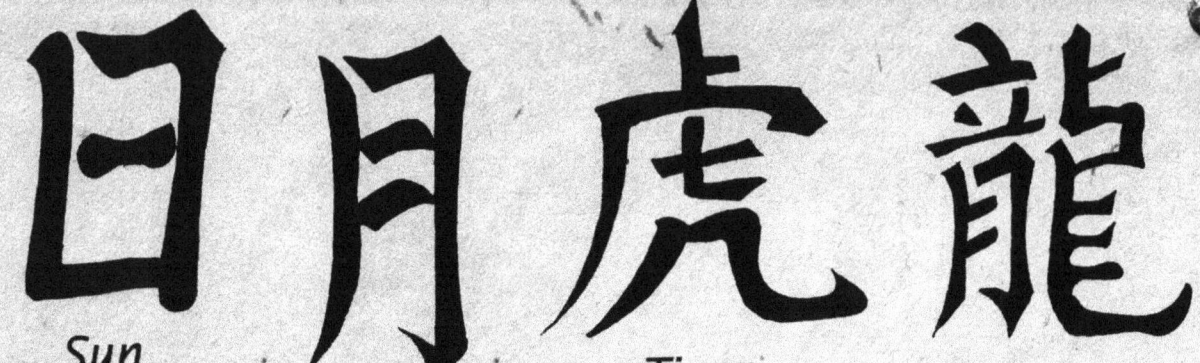

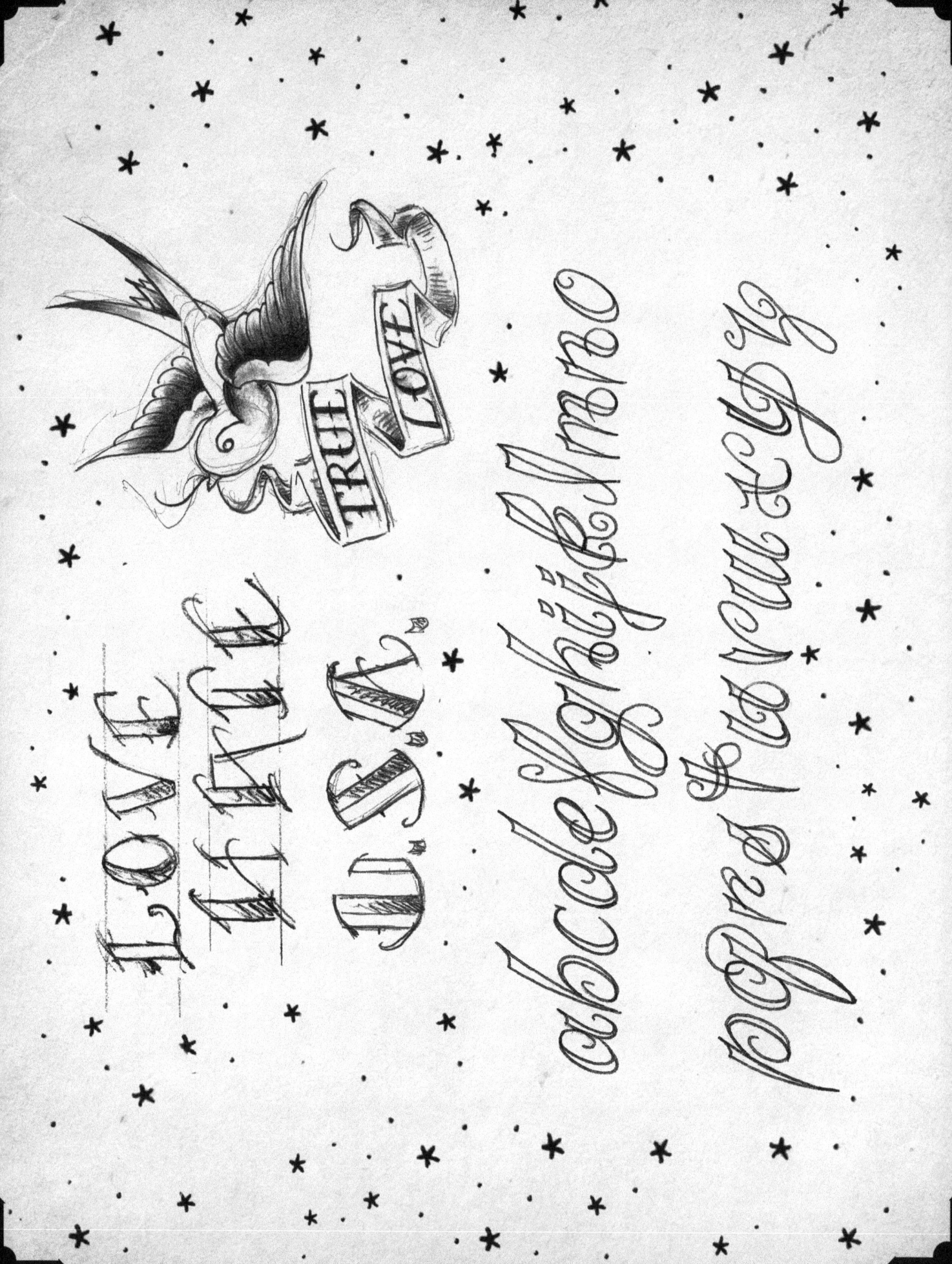

ABCDEFG
HIJKLM
NOPQRST
UVWXYZ

Live Strong

Live Strong

Live Strong

Live Strong

Live Strong

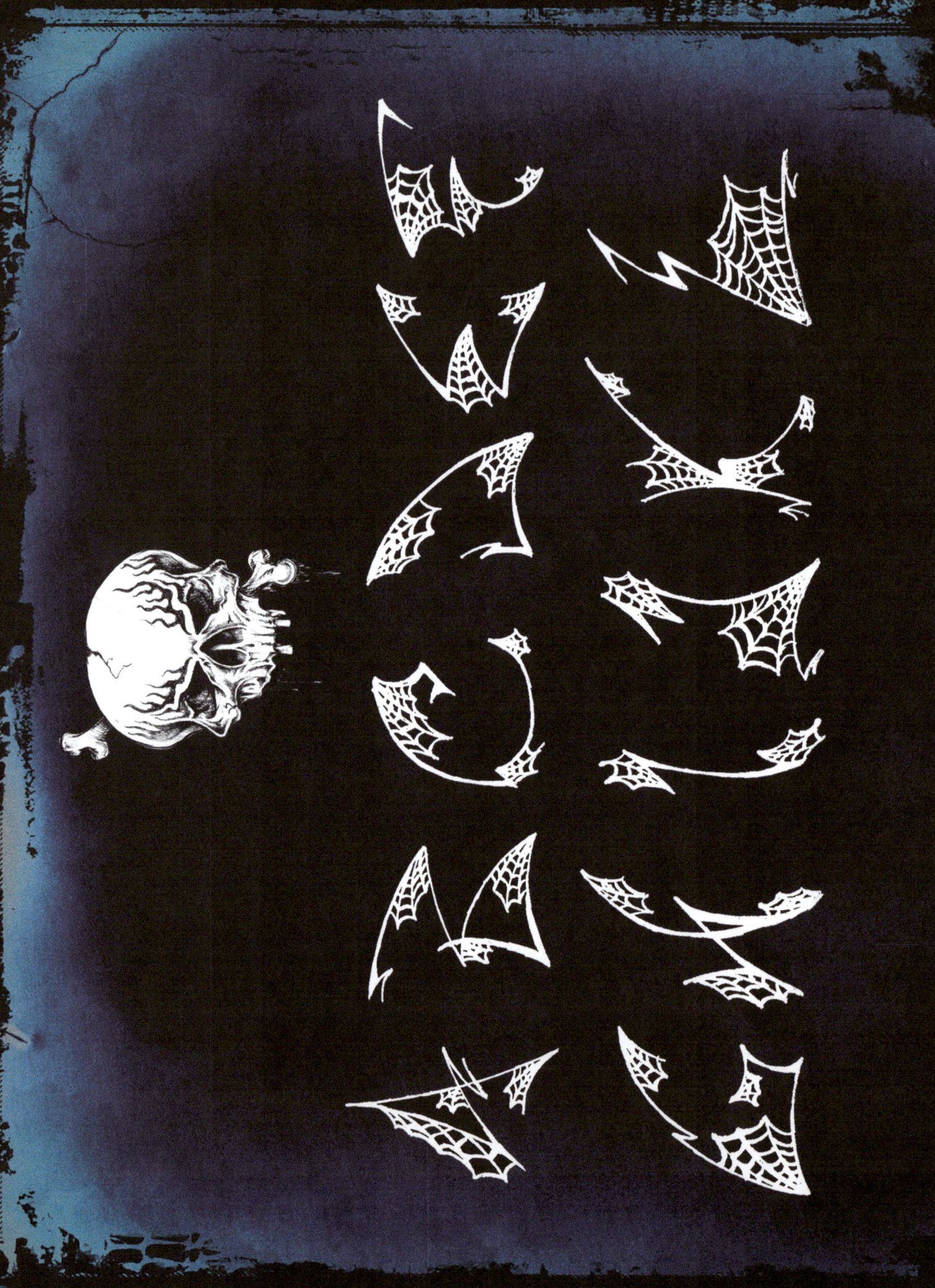

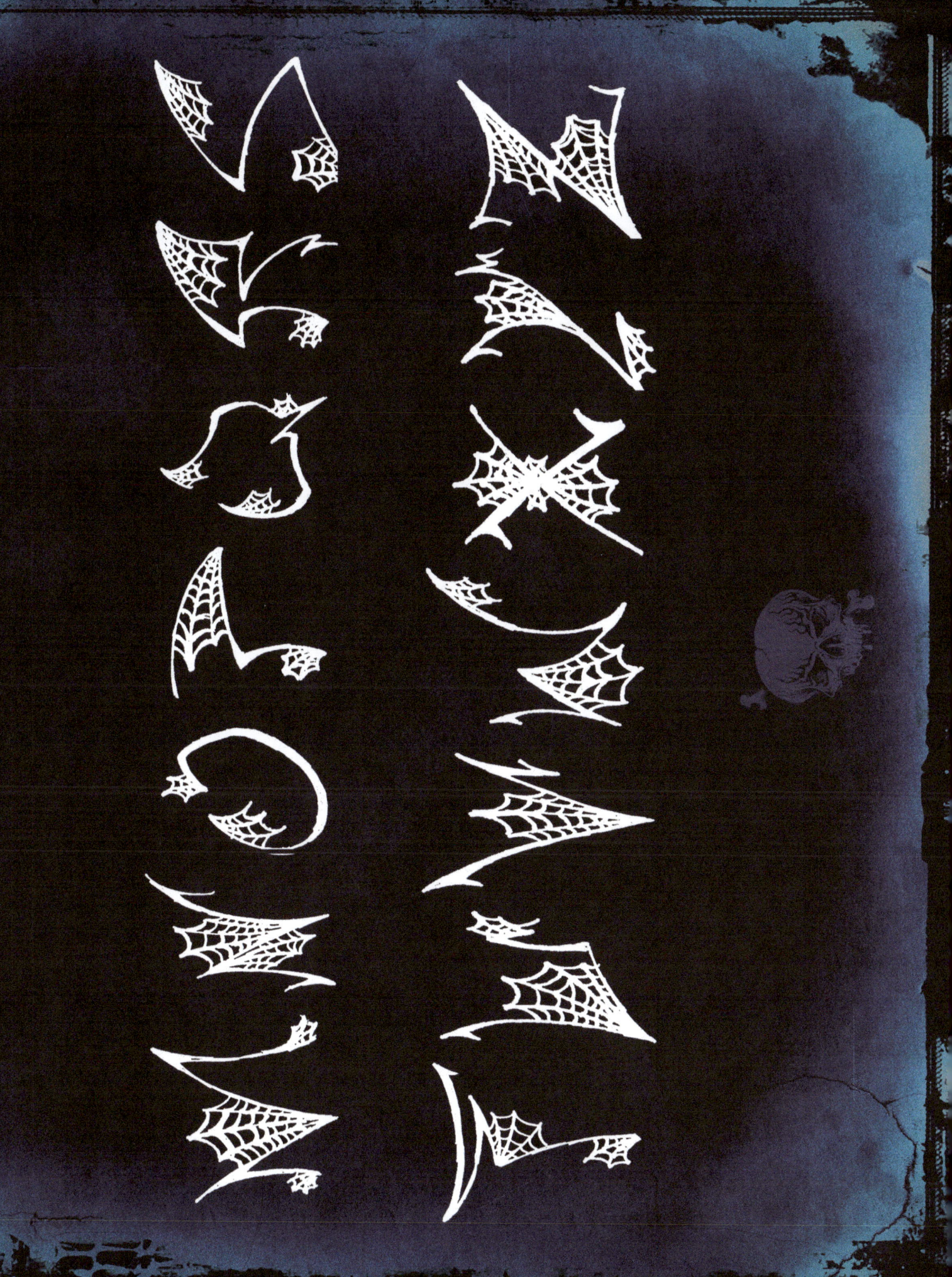

- Nothing Left To Lose
- Nothing Left To Lose
- Nothing Left To Lose
- Nothing Left To Lose

Victory

Victory   **VICTORY**   *Victory*

Victory   *Victory*   *Victory*

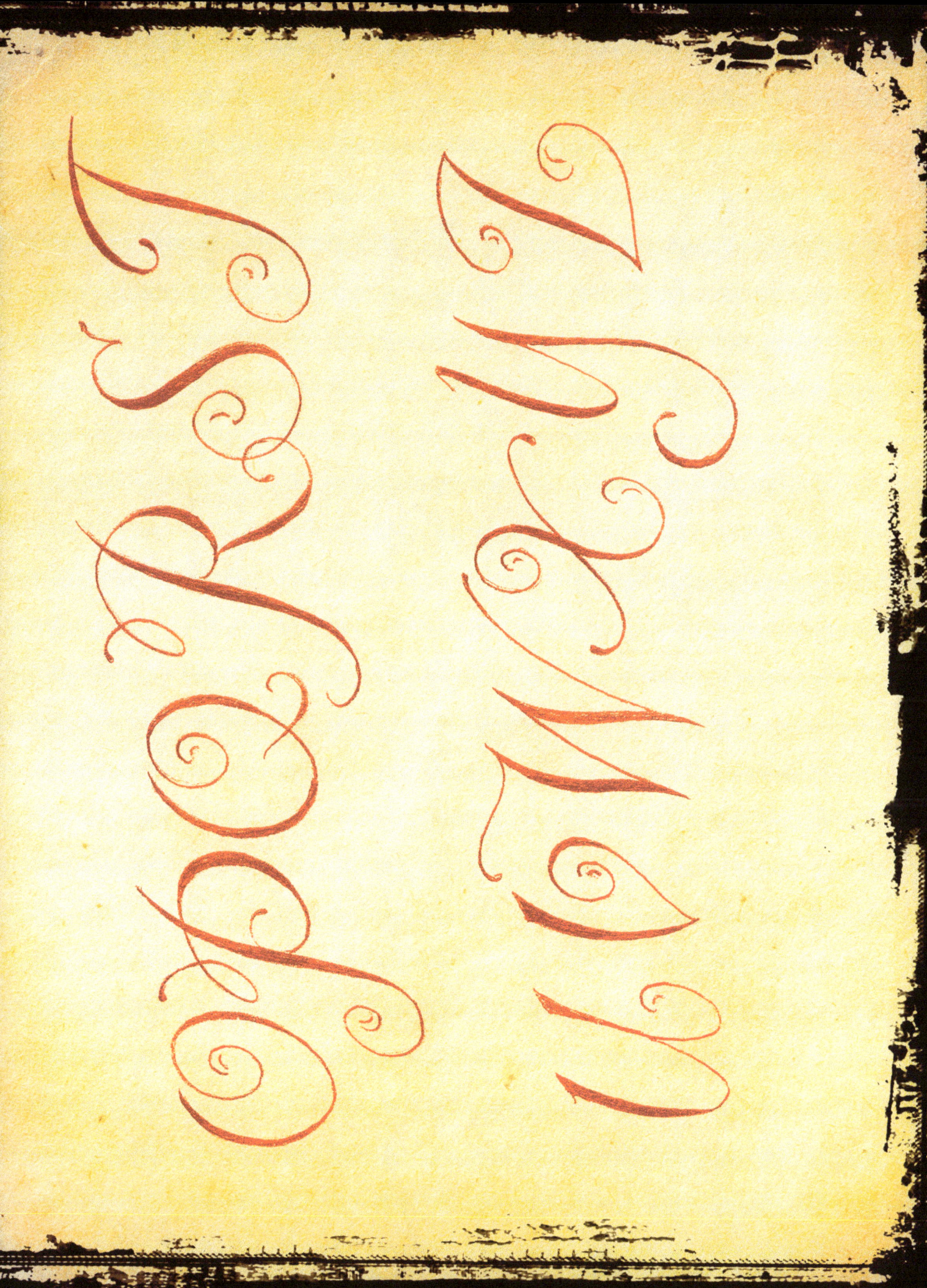

Beautiful

BEAUTIFUL

Beautiful

Beautiful

Beautiful

Beautiful

Only God Can Judge Me

Only God Can Judge Me

Only God Can Judge Me

Only God Can Judge Me

Peace

Peace

Peace

Peace

Peace

Peace

No Regrets

No Regrets

No Regrets

No Regrets

No Regrets

No Regrets

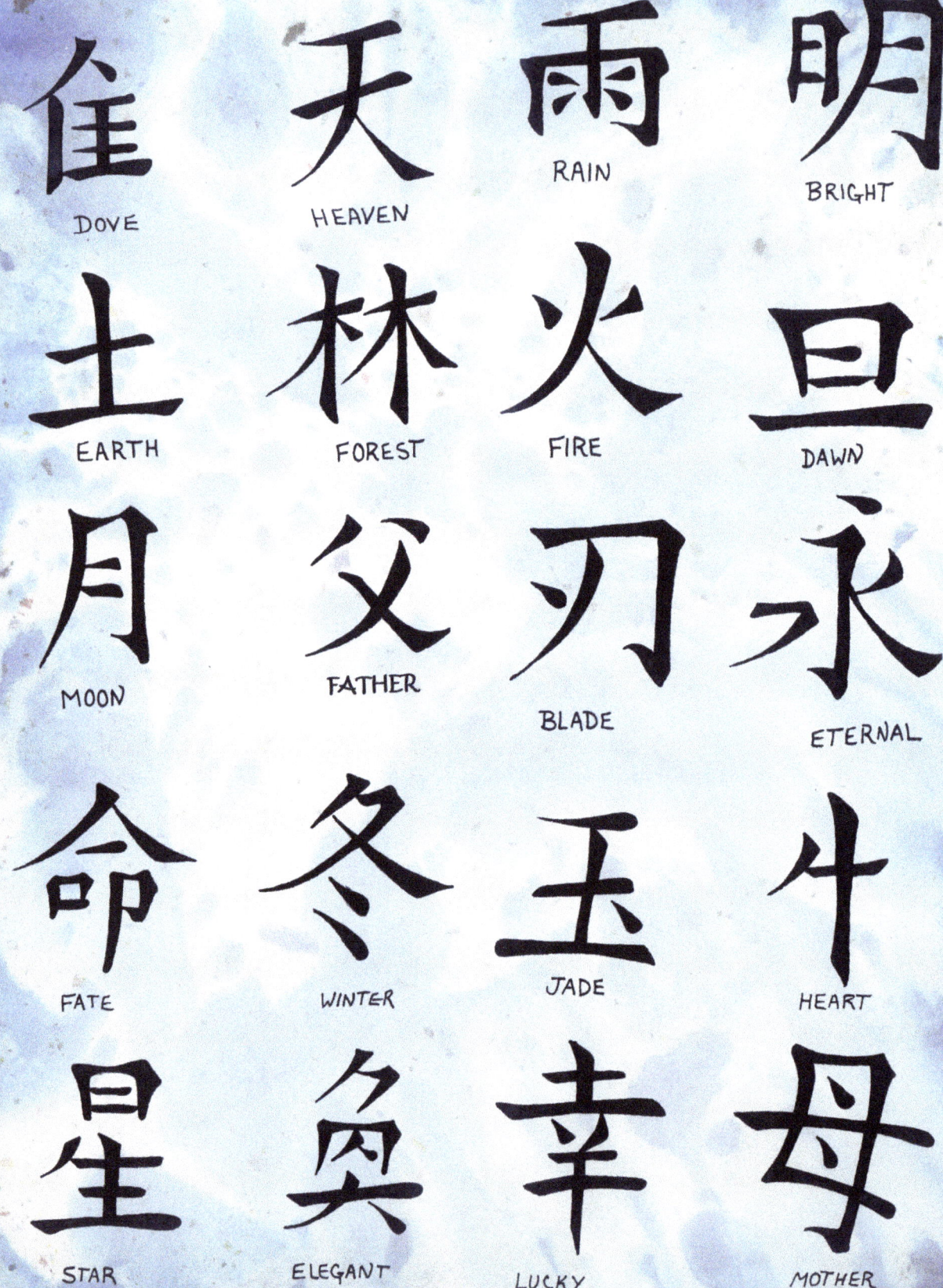

ABCDEFG
HIJKLMNO
OPQRSTU
VWXYZ

ABCDEFG
HIJKLMN
OPQRST
UVWXYZ

Tattoo Books
From ArtKulture & Superior Tattoo

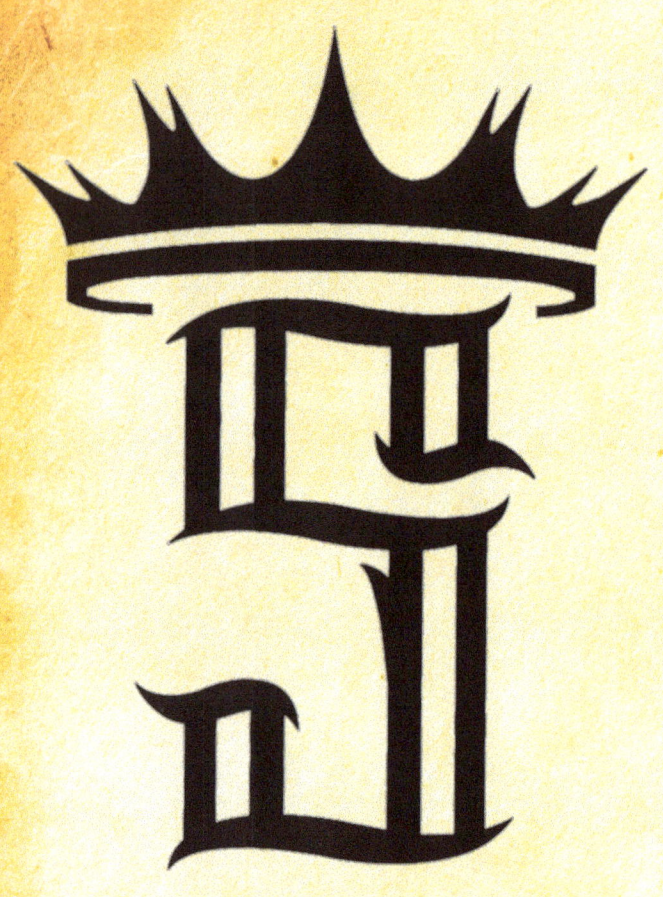

Tattoo Sketch Book
Author: Jim Watson
$32.95

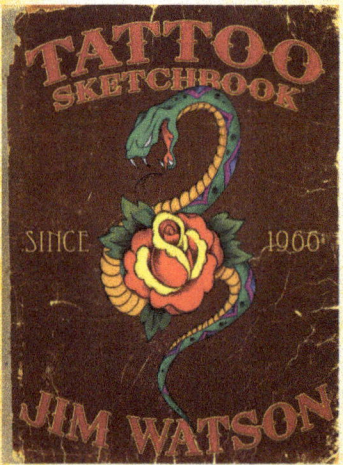

In recent years, the "tattoo artist sketchbook" has become a valuable resource for great tattoo ideas and designs. Although Jim Watson's tattoo style is normally recognized for being bright and colorful, these sketches show the reader the drawing technique and sketching process of a tattoo artist. The pages contain valuable reference sketches for tattoo artists, and is a great source for easy-to-copy, and easy-to-perform tattoo designs. For anyone who needs to tattoo a "Mom" across a traditional heart, or "Harley-Davidson" down someone's arm, Jim provides a variety or simple and elaborate "fonts" so you're sure to have the correct type style for a given situation. Produced on heavy paper with a hard cover, Jim's personal sketches are bound so the book lays flat on a table, all the better to fully study and utilize the numerous images. This collection will help everyone from new artists to journeymen; as well as their clients, to select (and, if needed, modify) the tattoo that they want and need.

Tattoo Bible Book One
Author: Superior Tattoo
$34.95

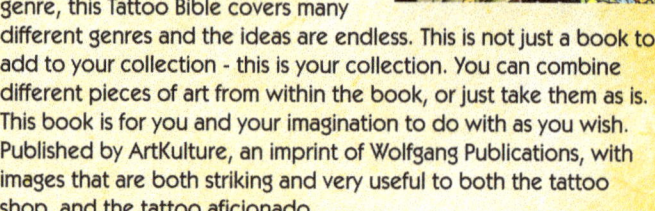

Whether you are preparing for your first tattoo or your twenty-seventh, you need artwork and designs that are just right. Tattoo Bible, authored by Superior Tattoo, provides well over 500 pieces of unique flash art - flash never before compiled into one single book.
While most tattoo books available today concentrate on one specific genre, this Tattoo Bible covers many different genres and the ideas are endless. This is not just a book to add to your collection - this is your collection. You can combine different pieces of art from within the book, or just take them as is. This book is for you and your imagination to do with as you wish. Published by ArtKulture, an imprint of Wolfgang Publications, with images that are both striking and very useful to both the tattoo shop, and the tattoo aficionado.

Tattoo Bible Book Two
Author: Superior Tattoo
$34.95

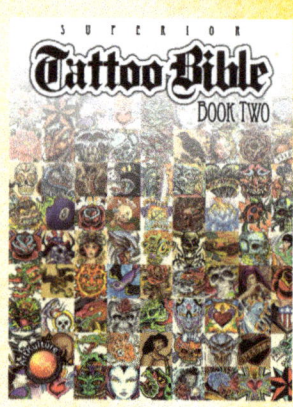

Based on the success of Book One, ArtKulture brings to market Tattoo Bible - Book Two, another unique and colorful collection of flash art. Everything is here, from Skulls to Tribal, Americana to the avant-garde.
Tattoo Bible includes a unique collection of new flash images from Superior's collection. The artists included in this book include the very well known, and those artists who should be well known. The best known names include Kevin LeBlanc, Aaron Coleman, Bob Sims, Nate Powers and many, many more.
Tattoo Bible - Book Two, covers different styles and an endless supply of ideas. Make your own design by combining different pieces of art from within the book, or use one of the images as a stand-alone tattoo. Book Two, includes over 500 pieces of flash art. Colorful tattoo images that are useful to both the tattoo shop, and the tattoo aficionado.

Tattoo Bible Book Three
Author: Superior Tattoo
$34.95

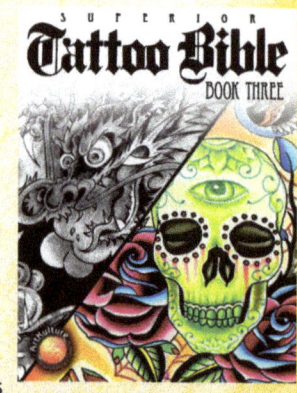

Book Three, the newest installment in the popular Superior Tattoo Bible series, continues the tradition of offering a vast collection of only the best tattoo artwork available.
Unlike the earlier Bibles, Tattoo Bible Book Three is a collection of designs from opposite ends of the spectrum. This new book contains images from both the old school and the new.
With over 350 images, this new book is the perfect companion for any tattooist, from the aspiring novice to the seasoned vet; and a useful resource for tattoo aficionados looking for the art they need to create the ultimate tattoo design. Book Three showcases artwork from some of the most-recognizable names in the tattoo world, as well as the coolest, trendiest designs from some of the newest, up-and-coming talent in the industry! Whether you're an artist or enthusiast, this book will become an essential tool for years to come!